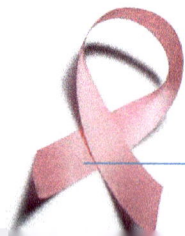

Her Story

The Legacy of Her Fight

The Devotional

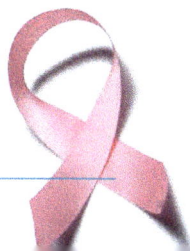

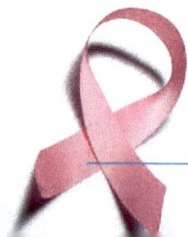

Her Story

The Legacy of Her Fight

The Devotional

By

Minister Onedia N. Gage

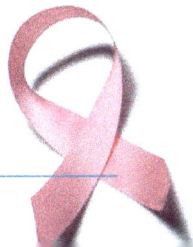

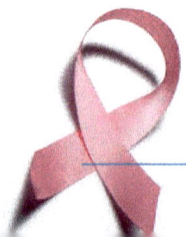

More Books by Minister Onedia N. Gage

Are You Ready for 9th Grade . . . Again? A Family's Guide to Success
As We Grow Together for Expectant Couples Bible Study Her Workbook
As We Grow Together for Expectant Couples Bible Study His Workbook
As We Grow Together for Expectant Couples Daily Devotional
As We Grow Together for Expectant Couples Prayer Journal
The Best 40 Days of Your Life: A Journey of Spiritual Renewal
The Blue Print: Poetry for the Soul
From Two to One: The Notebook for the Christian Couple
Hannah's Voice: Powerful Lessons in Prayer
Her Story, The Legacy of Her Fight: The Legacy Journal
Her Story, The Legacy of Her Fight: Prayers and Journal
ILY! A Mother Daughter Relationship Workbook
In Her Own Words: Notebook for the Christian Woman
In Purple Ink: Poetry for the Spirit
The Intensive Retreat for Couples for Her
The Intensive Retreat for Couples for Him
Living a Whole Life: Sermons which Promote, Prompt and Provoke Life
Love Letters to God from a Teenage Girl
The Measure of a Woman: The Details of Her Soul
The Notebook: For Me, About Me, By Me
The Notebook for the Christian Teen
On This Journey Daily Devotional for Young People
On This Journey Prayer Journal for Young People
On This Journey Prayer Journal for Young People, Vol. 2
One Day More Than We Deserve Prayer Journal for the Growing Christian
Promises, Promises: A Christian Novel
Tools for These Times: Timely Sermons for Uncertain Times
Walking Tall With a Broken Life
With An Anointed Voice: The Power of Prayer
Yielded and Submitted: A Woman's Journey for a Life Dedicated to God
Yielded and Submitted: A Woman's Journey for a Life Dedicated to God Intimate Study
Yielded and Submitted: A Woman's Journey for a Life Dedicated to God Prayers and
Journal

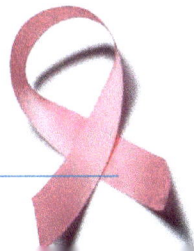

Library of Congress

Her Story: The Legacy of Her Fight

The Devotional

Purple Ink, Inc. Press

For Information:
Purple Ink, Inc.
P O Box 300113
Houston, TX 77230

www.purpleink.net ♦ onediagage@purpleink.net

www.onediagage.com ♦ onediagage@onediagage.com

ISBN:

978-1-939119-49-0

Printed in United States

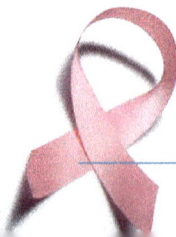

Dedication

To the women who are in this fight

To the women who will fight

To the women who have succumbed to the fight

To the time she spends with God

To the man who holds her hand

To the children who are part of this fight without their knowledge or consent

To the community she serves and that supports her

To the people who are affected by her fight

To the people who work so that there is no fight necessary

To the legacy which while result because she is in the fight

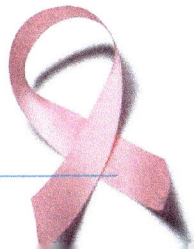

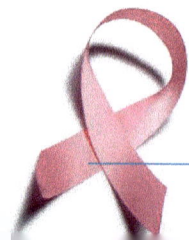

God's Words

Colossians 4:2 (NIV)

[2] Devote yourselves to prayer, being watchful and thankful.

Job 11:13 (NIV)

[13] "Yet if you devote your heart to Him and stretch out your hands to Him,

Romans 12:10 (NIV)

[10] Be devoted to one another in love. Honor one another above yourselves.

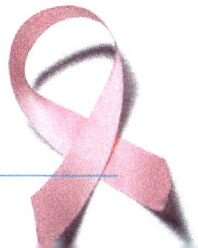

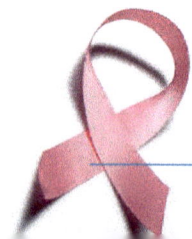

Dear God,

I pray You bless the women whose lives are affected by this disease. I pray that because this has occurred in their lives, with Your full knowledge and consent, that You let them know why they were chosen and trusted with this message.

Lord, allow them to see the need to help others survive the overall trauma of the event, but also be able to see Your beauty and Your splendor because of this illness.

Lord, remind her that her testimony serves You. Lord, keep her focused on You and hold her close in her despair and discomfort.

Lord, as she travels through her heart, mind, and spirit, I pray that You show her how she will bless, and therefore, serve others.

Lord, thank You for entrusting me with this book, these words, and this legacy. I pray that I listen to Your voice to share the correct words that You want seen. Lord, thank You for using me! Lord, I so want to impress You by obeying You!

I pray for these blessings in Jesus' name.

Amen.

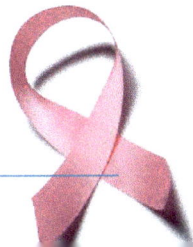

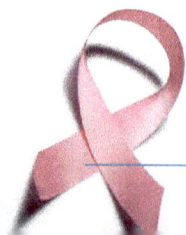

Dear Woman:

So you received what could easily be the worst news EVER but you are still here—STANDING! So now what? Well, you are holding this book, so you have started living and you have started healing.

My prayer is that your healing is instrumental and inspirational to others whose paths you will cross. In the meantime, as you study these devotionals, I hope that you also allow these words to minister to you so that you are whole emotionally and spiritually—better than ever before.

Use these pages to address your authentic self in an outlandish manner. You are a bold, courageous, trustworthy, and special woman. You have a message and now a cause, and a ministry. Let this time be spent seeking God for all that He is and all that He wants for you.

One of my favorite Bible verses is 1 Corinthians 13:13, the Message version, which reads: "Love extravagantly." This is a great time for you to remove the boundaries of your love and love bodaciously and with an understanding that you can NEVER run out. You are not the supplier of your own love. God is. Love because He loves you.

Further, love heals. In this love and healing, you can overcome. Use this time to heal from everything.

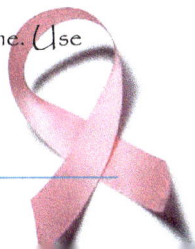

Surrender it all to God like you have never done before.

I pray for your wholeness. Wellness. Spirit. Love. Mission. Vision. Dreams. And achievements. This is part of your legacy. What you do next is more important than what happened. What happened should cause something BIG to happen next. Don't block the BIG! It is the best part of you!

Leave a HUGE legacy! Start with yourself!!

I look forward to hearing from you. Feel free to share with me as you journey. You can follow me on twitter @onediangage, email onediagage@onediagage.com, facebook.com/onediagageministries, blogtalkradio.com/onediagage, and youtube.com/onediagage.

I can hardly wait!

In His Service!

Onedia N. Gage

www.onediagage.com

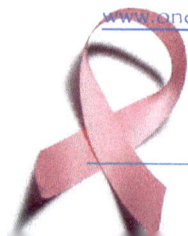

Instructions for use

♦ This is written in God's voice, so know that you He is talking to you.

♦ These are tools your journey.

♦ Read in any order you need.

♦ It is designed to be portable, used while you are waiting and healing.

♦ The devotional can be used daily and repeatedly.

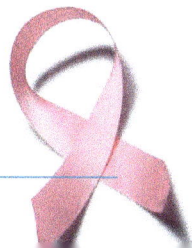

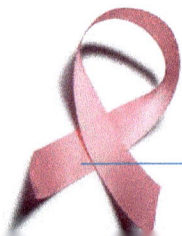

Table of Contents

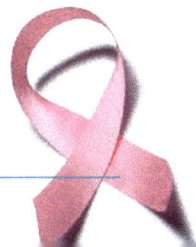

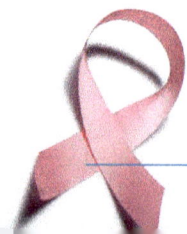

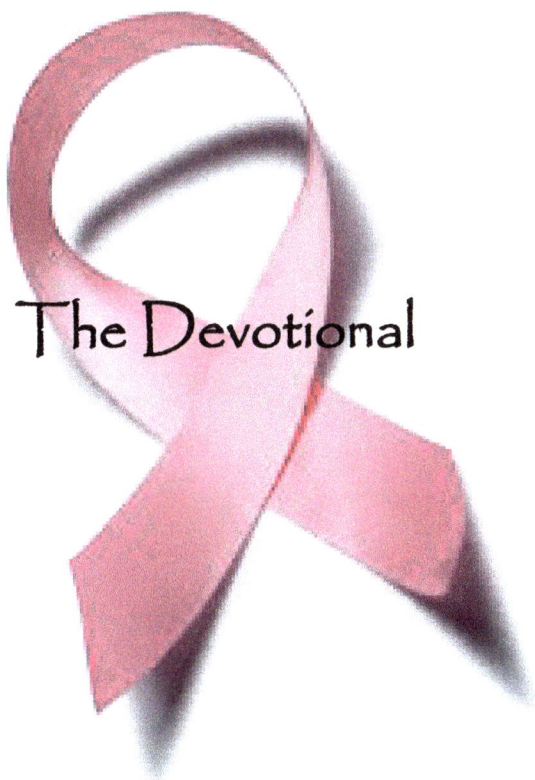

The Devotional

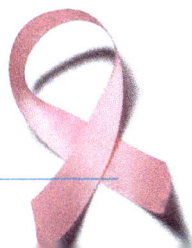

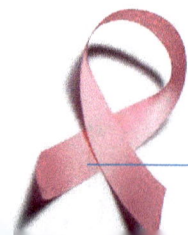

Genesis 2:21-22 (NIV) [21] So the LORD God caused the man to fall into a deep sleep; and while he was sleeping, he took one of the man's ribs and then closed up the place with flesh. [22] Then the LORD God made a woman from the rib he had taken out of the man, and he brought her to the man.

I created you.

When I planned the world, I had you in mind. I thought of you as I created the Earth. I considered what you would do in response to My Earth. I knew what you would like, what type of parents and family you have, and what makes you smile.

I created you so I know your every move, your every thought, your every action, and not to mention your next attitude. I am your God because I created you.

I allow you to make decisions but that does **NOT** allow you to leave and distance yourself from Me.

I created you so automatically I love you. I created you so I know your moods and your laughter. I know the meaning of your tears. I know you will still sin in a certain area.

I created you and I know all about you. Because I created you, I love you. I also forgive you. I teach you. I provide for you. I give you gifts. I invested within you with gifts. I give you the opportunity to share those gifts with others in order to bring Me glory. I created you. Not for the amusement of Myself but for My glory.

I created you for My purposes. I created you to serve Me. I created you to help others to know Me.

I created you to love. Me and everybody else.

I created you.

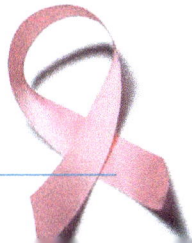

Jeremiah 1:5 (NIV) [5] "Before I formed you in the womb I knew you, before you were born I set you apart; I appointed you as a prophet to the nations."

I knew you first.

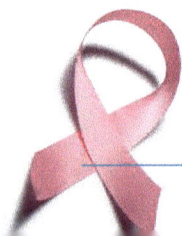

I created you so I knew you first. I know you better than you know yourself, so I definitely know you better than your family and friends do. I am intentional about the details I have placed into you and how I have built you.

I knew you first. I know aspects that you will never share and some of which you will not understand.

I knew you first, which means that all others, including you, are second in knowledge and understanding and love and all other details.

I continue to know you best. I continue to understand you better than you understand yourself. I continue to keep you whole. I am your God. Your Creator. Your Forgiver. I am your Peace Keeper. Peacemaker. I know what you need daily. Hourly. Daily. Weekly. Monthly. Yearly.

I give you permission to put your attitude down because you don't think I know you or remember you or your needs. I provide you with everything you need at the time you need it. We do not measure that need or those supplies the same but I do have your best interest, according to My will, in mind.

So relax, Daughter. I am here for you as you are here for Me.

Please stop fretting over what others say and do, understand and do not understand. They are not supposed to understand. They do not even understand themselves, so why are you expecting them to understand you?

I knew you first.

Jeremiah 29:11 (NIV) [11] For I know the plans I have for you," declares the LORD, "plans to prosper you and not to harm you, plans to give you hope and a future.

I have plans for you.

Child, when I created you, I had plans for you! As your God, I am able to override whatever plans you have developed for yourself. My plans for you are according to My will—My sovereign, auspicious will! You do not know all of My will and you do not understand the elements of My will.

My will for your life is far greater than you can ever imagine and I gave you that imagination. What I hope you will do is trust Me. Remember I planned you. I created your conception. I got you here. You lived when you could have died. I spared your life when the odds of you being born were slim. I birthed you and they wanted to put you in the NICU, but you never went. You survived that disease and that infection and that allergy.

You got that job but your qualifications were short. You wanted one job but got a different one that you liked better that actually did not exist until you needed it.

I have plans for you that you will know only when I manifest them into existence. I developed these plans based on My vision for you. I have plans for you that even you will envy.

I have plans for you which require you to remain faithful and steadfast in me. I require that you keep Me first. At all times. I have plans for you. Just keep in mind that I am here always. My plans will happen.

Trust. Belief. Faith.

My plans will always override yours.

My plans include all of your issues and conditions.

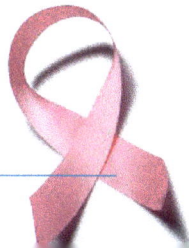

Ephesians 3:18-19 (NIV) [18] may have power, together with all the Lord's holy people, to grasp how wide and long and high and deep is the love of Christ, [19] and to know this love that surpasses knowledge—that you may be filled to the measure of all the fullness of God.

I love you.

I love you! I created you! So why wouldn't I love you?! You keep questioning Me about loving you. I love you! You are going to be older when you understand the love I love with. I love you truly unconditionally and with an infinity matched by none other.

When I gave Paul those words, he could write and preach and believe those words because I had loved him even through his persecution of Me to his transformation because of Me.

When you consider the length, depth, width and height of any physical object, there are measurements attached to that figure which allows you to calculate the area, perimeter, volume, surface are, and the lateral surface area. However, when you look at the dimensions of My love, you cannot measure My love numerically because the manner in which I love you cannot be duplicated by yourself or others. My love is indefinite! My love is infinite!

I love you when you don't love yourself. I consider My love the most authentic aspect of your life. My love is the only thing that you can really depend on. My love is the only love that you have which is unconditional, unlimited, and unconventional. Keep in mind, you don't even think that you deserve My love.

My love keeps you sane, keeps you focused, keeps you grounded, keeps you out of the enemy's hands, and keeps you humble. My love keeps you alive. My love keeps you out of trouble. My love helps you sleep at night. You would go crazy in your own spirit, but because of My love you are sane, whole and healthy.

I love you! My love gives you the power to move when you can't. My love gives you the energy to persevere when you really want to quit. My love sustains you and lifts you and refines you and elevates you when you need it the most.

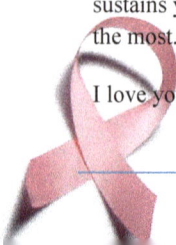

I love you!

John 7:5 (NIV) [5] For even his own brothers did not believe in him.

I believe in you!

I believe in you! I created you! I have a plan where I planned things for you so My believing in you is critical. Why wouldn't I believe in you? I put you in those places where you would be questioned and disbelieved. I need to believe in you because I trust you to do the things I planned. I believe in you to carry out My plans for you.

If I didn't believe in you or trust you, I could have given that assignment to someone else. I could have given that gift to someone else.

I believe in you when you doubt but you should not. I believe in you because I have given you the tools to do the task. I believe in you because I have placed people in your path and your reach to help you achieve what I designed you to do. I believe in you because you asked Me to enlarge your territory at a time when you had achieved the first of the plans that I had for you. Because you had done as I instructed, I enlarged your territory. This belief is not wasted on you. I am heavily invested in you and your life.

I believe in you and if you don't quit, I will see you through all that I have planned for you.

Stop doubting your abilities. I gave them to you. Stop questioning why you. The answer is because I said so. Stop trying to quit on the assignments which I have planned and designed. I designed these gifts, talents, and projects for you so I know what you are capable of. I did not give you anything that you are not capable of.

I believe in you and when you doubt, you demonstrate that you do not trust Me!

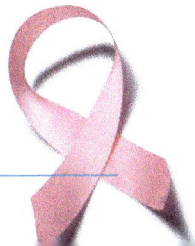

Proverbs 2:6 (NIV) [6] For the LORD gives wisdom; from his mouth come knowledge and understanding.

I gave you wisdom!

I am the only One who can give you wisdom and allow you wisdom as a result of your experiences. Wisdom is produced from your experiences. I am the Sole Author of that.

The problem I have with 'wise' people is often they are wise in their own eyes rather than in My eyes. I equip you with wisdom to ultimately serve Me. Wisdom I give is often misused for the personal good of those who I have gifted to possess it. But rather I granted you wisdom to serve Me through others. I have people that I need to send your way who need the lessons which you have experienced, but that wisdom is not to be used selectively. If someone comes to you with the details that offer you an opportunity to share your testimony and the lessons you have learned and the wisdom that you have acquired, then assume that I sent them and share so that they can get what I sent them for.

Wisdom should lead you to want to help others—wisdom is not to be used to keep Me away from others because they do not meet your approval. Remember, wisdom means that you did not even meet your own approval at one point. You started meeting your own approval because of the wisdom that I provide.

Wisdom is to be used wisely but not sparingly. I gave you wisdom to use. I did not limit your wisdom or your access to wisdom. I also did not give you the power to withhold it from others.

Wisdom is not wisdom if you keep it to yourself.

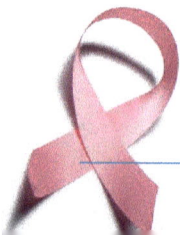

Matthew 6:15 (NIV) [15] But if you do not forgive others their sins, your Father will not forgive your sins.

I want you to forgive.

I want you to forgive others who harm you or whatever you are holding that grudge for. If I remember the situation correctly, I blessed you with some things that you asked for after that. Why do you find value in withholding forgiveness? What do you gain? Anything? What satisfaction do you get by remembering the worst mistake a person has ever made toward you? Why do you retell that same story over and over again, even when nobody's listening? Don't you think I would fill that space with more of My love if you could let that issue go? Do you know that the other person does not think about it like you do? Do you know that you gain nothing by your unforgiveness?

The fact of the matter is that by not forgiving others, you hold your own self hostage. That hostage behavior keeps you in a dark place, where I cannot even reach you. When you don't forgive others, you demonstrate that you don't believe in Me. I heal you when you others hurt you. When I heal you, forgive them. I bless you when they hurt you. I bless you, forgive them. I created both of you. Neither of you are perfect and neither are without faults. I am working with both of you.

When you forgive, you grow. You learn to release the things that don't matter in the grand scheme. When you forgive, you have surrendered to Me in the ultimate way—one that yields the best blessings and gives the best benefits.

I know that forgiveness is harder at times than others, but take refuge in Me. I am the Great I Am. I am your Strong Tower. I am your Forgiver, which makes forgiving very valuable.

Forgive just because I said so.

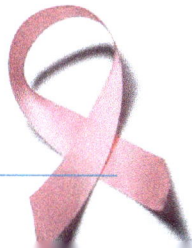

Psalm 42:9 (NIV) [9] I say to God my Rock, "Why have you forgotten me? Why must I go about mourning, oppressed by the enemy?"

I have not forgotten about you.

I know it may seem like I am not present because I am not giving you everything you asked for or that you are having difficulties in life. However, I am right here. I am your God. I have never abandoned not one of my children. Even when they have done some of the most deplorable things. Remember what Cain did to Able? I still spoke to Cain, protected Cain and chastised Cain for being wrong.

I did not forget Joseph when he was serving Pharaoh. I took his story full circle, and because he was faithful, honorable, and forgiving during his period of exile, I restored him to his family. He served them as if nothing happened. Joseph's attitude was phenomenal.

Realize that when I am silent, I may be requiring you to remember, recall and reflect on your lessons which I have already taught you but you opted out of using.

I have some things I want you to do when you are convinced that I have forgotten you:

- Read My word—the Bible
- Listen to My voice—I have said things to you that because you were so focused on your own thoughts that you missed My message of comfort and peace.
- Recall all of the times when I gave you exactly what you ask for and you still wanted more.
- Recall the times I did not give you what you asked for and you are still grateful for what I saved you from.
- Remember all of things you thought would distance us but did not.
- I have not forgotten you! I will never forget you!

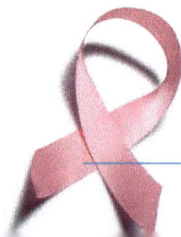

John 3:16 (NIV) [16] For God so loved the world that He gave His one and only Son, that whoever believes in Him shall not perish but have eternal life.

I gave up more than you ever will.

When I birthed the universe and all of its contents, I knew what would happen to My creation. I knew then what you have come to learn now: you need a Saviour. So it was My Son whom I choose to save you and everyone else from all of the consequences, including My consequences. Yes, it was painful for Me. I didn't want to do that but I know everyone that I have created.

When you complain, whine even, about what you are experiencing and enduring and what happened, remember you would not have given up your child. No matter what I said to you, you would not have willingly given up your child, which I blessed you to conceive and birth, to save anyone—possibly not even yourself.

I love you which is why I gave you My saving grace—My Son. Jesus' blood was shed for you! He asked Me several times to remove that job from Him but I said no. My will be done. Could I have changed My mind? Sure, I could have, but the entire world would have to change.

I planned His birth for thousands of years. I only allowed Him to walk this earth for 33 years. Jesus never sinned. Jesus did ALL that I asked of Him. You think it's hard to be your parent or your child. What do you think He felt?

I gave up a lot! The most actually. I gave up everything. I did gain Him with Me in Heaven, so consider carefully how you would feel if you were Mary. First, there was the ridicule of being pregnant without a husband. Then I took Our Son and they crucified Him on a cross. Such pain. So many questions.

I am God and God alone. I want better for you than you even know to want for yourself.

I love you enough to save you. Daily.

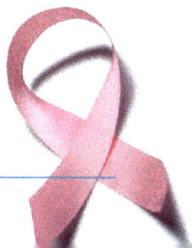

Job 1:8-12 (NIV) [8] Then the LORD said to Satan, "Have you considered my servant Job? There is no one on earth like him; he is blameless and upright, a man who fears God and shuns evil." [9] "Does Job fear God for nothing?" Satan replied. [10] "Have you not put a hedge around him and his household and everything he has? You have blessed the work of his hands, so that his flocks and herds are spread throughout the land. [11] But now stretch out your hand and strike everything he has, and he will surely curse you to your face." [12] The LORD said to Satan, "Very well, then, everything he has is in your power, but on the man himself do not lay a finger." Then Satan went out from the presence of the LORD.

I chose you out of My trust for you.

Noah. David. Boaz. Hannah. Joseph. Mary. Paul. Jesus. Samuel. Abraham. Esther. Mordecai. Job. This is not comprehensive list and it is in no particular order of people I trusted and had their stories written in the Bible. While there is not a Bible to publish your story in, I am building a story for you to share because I trust you.

I invest in you and equip you with the same tools that they had. I am disappointed when you do not use those tools, you quit, give up and resign; you consider My assignments beneath you and you only praise Me when what I provide in on your list, rather than what is in My will.

Others know My level of protection for you and My love for you. Others envy the favor I have for you. You may not always realize it but I do.

I have to trust you for you to fully benefit from My will. I need you to understand My investment and My promises are comparable. I am always going to protect you. I am not going to let anyone hurt you.

Put your hand back in My hand and rest there.

My trust, protection, and love.

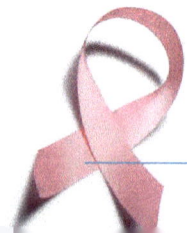

Acts 9:4 (NIV) [4] He fell to the ground and heard a voice say to him, "Saul, Saul, why do you persecute me?"

I am in charge of your path.

Child, I know that I gave you freedom of speech, an imagination, a mind, an intellect that I empowered you to educate, and a drive to do it all—at the same time, but I want to remind you that I am still in charge of you and your path!

I open and close doors. I put you in the places that I want you to be in. I can get your attention however I please.

I called Samuel out of his sleep. I stopped Saul in his tracks. I brought Naomi back home. I gave Elizabeth a child. I equipped Noah to build an ark. These are details that they never thought would exist, however, I did that by directing their path.

Once you realize that I know what happens next, what the motives of other persons are, what you need, and how all of these pieces work together.

Remember that when you avoid My will or question the path I provide, you attempt to delay My will. Consider Saul who I transformed into Paul, who preached 10 days after I blinded Saul on the road. Paul went on to preach, teach, mentor, and pray. And penned almost half of the New Testament.

There is a reason that I am in charge. I have saved you from some of the absolutely worse mistakes ever. All because you were trying to stray from My path. If I can put Saul-turned-Paul on the right path, why can't you trust Me to do the same for you?

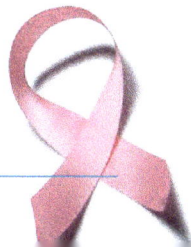

Psalm 46:1 (NIV) [1] God is our refuge and strength, an ever-present help in trouble.

I am your refuge.

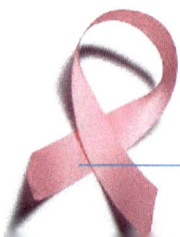

I am your refuge. Your safe place to land, your safe haven. I am your hiding place. Your go-to. Your survival kit. I am your Source. Your strength. Your place of solace. Your place of solitude. I am your refuge! You can meltdown with Me, tell Me anything and everything, even though it's embarrassing. I already know anyway. I am your safe place—the Only One you have.

Why do I have to tell you this?

Why do I have to keep reminding you of this?

Remember when you were ill, I was there. Remember, I got you that job which you didn't really qualify for. Remember, I dried your tears at that funeral. I picked you up after the divorce. I kept you children safe when the senseless gun violence took the lives of several children and teachers. I kept you form the 9/11 attacks. I reached out for you when you walked away because you thought I had left you.

I really do everything to keep you inaccessible to your go-to's which cause you to sin.

I want you to come to Me when you are down or depressed, sad or sorry, burdened or blamed, bowed or broken, aggravated or angry.

Me. I. Your God.

I am here and I want you to seek Me for what you need and keeping you whole. Most importantly, keeping you accessible to Me. I will prevent your 'stuff' from interfering with our relationship.

I am your refuge.

1 Peter 2:9 (NIV) [9] But you are a chosen people, a royal priesthood, a holy nation, God's special possession, that you may declare the praises of him who called you out of darkness into his wonderful light.

I chose you.

This is not something that just happened to you. I chose you. I chose you because of the people who will need you and that those will come into your path will need to understand your situation to comprehend what they will face personally.

I choose you! You are not My back-up plan or second choice. I do not have someone that is just on standby to do your job.

I choose you! So do your job. Do your assignment. Be obedient. Stop shirking your responsibilities. Stop hiding. Quit your excuses. You have no real reason for fear. I am here. This is My plan—not something that you thought up.

I choose you like so many others, actually everybody, to do a job which furthers My kingdom and helps others to confess Me, love Me, and know Me. That is everyone's base calling and talent.

I choose you and I do not make mistakes. I do not make decisions which do not produce My desired result. I have not made a mistake in anything I have done and never will.

Just for your information: you are not a mistake your parents made either. I know that is what they think but your birth was planned—by Me.

I choose you—don't let Me down.

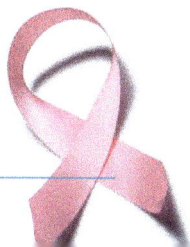

Psalm 46:10 (NIV) [10] He says, "Be still, and know that I am God; I will be exalted among the nations, I will be exalted in the earth."

I am your God.

I am your God. This is hard to handle most of the time because the world I created gets out of hand. I am in competition with others and material things which I allowed to be created.

I am important to you because I created you, I know you, and I have plans. I cannot be replaced by anyone or anything. I am a jealous God. I am that I am. The Great I Am. I know that you don't always keep Me first and that is a problem as well. I consider you one of My best works but your responses and behavior does not speak to that.

I am your God, I am accessible to you. I am attentive to you. I am responsive to you. I keep you safe and protected. I keep the hedge of protection around you high—really high. I talk to you. I answer your prayers. I give you blessings that you don't deserve.

Yet, I am still behind everyone else. And everything else. It is not what I deserve. I brought you to Me when you had walked away from Me after that disappointment but I took her. I found you when you were damaged and broken and hurting. I am your God. Because I Am, you are happier, more complete, more whole.

I am your God! I am on watch. I am right here. I need your attention to help you. I know that being still is a difficult concept but absolutely necessary.

I am your God! I do not need <u>any</u> help!

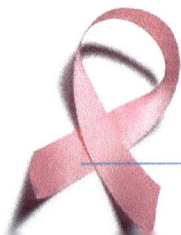

Matthew 11:28-30 (NIV) [28] "Come to Me, all you who are weary and burdened, and I will give you rest. [29] Take My yoke upon you and learn from me, for I am gentle and humble in heart, and you will find rest for your souls. [30] For My yoke is easy and My burden is light."

I am your burden bearer.

I know that you have burdens. I know what your burdens are. I know that some of those burdens are optional.

Shed the burdens, all of them. I want you to strongly consider the weight which will be lifted so that you have more time, energy, and desire to serve Me. So here is the road map on where to start so that can eliminate the burdens from your life: things that you don't control—which is everything! Specifically, that job, any job, money, kids, people that do not invest in you, and people in general.

I will hear everything that you have on your heart, mind and soul. I have never closed My ears to you. When you share your burdens with Me, I do have some expectations. When you give Me your burdens, leave the burdens alone. Once I have it, let it go! Don't keep your hand on it. Don't keep your mind on it. Don't keep talking about it. And please don't keep worrying about it.

If I have it, then that means you have more time for Me.

The burdens that keep you from loving Me, or serving Me, or following Me, are the burdens that I want!

I bear them. Give them over.

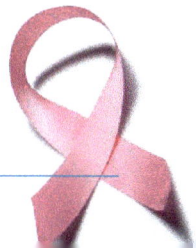

John 14:15-17 (NIV) [15] "If you love Me, keep My commands. [16] And I will ask the Father, and He will give you another advocate to help you and be with you forever— [17] the Spirit of truth. The world cannot accept Him, because it neither sees Him nor knows Him. But you know Him, for He lives with you and will be in you.

I left you with a Comforter.

I told you that My Father, God, would give you a comforter—the Holy Spirit to help you through your days—your good ones but mostly your bad days.

I gave you that Comforter because you were going to have some devastating days. You were going to cry for help. In My infinite wisdom, I provided you with a Comforter, pre-disaster, pre-catastrophic, pre-health issues, pre-unemployment, pre-everything. The Comforter is provided for you so that you can walk away from those elements which result in sin. You need to seek the Comforter because the sins you selected are so detrimental and they still require to seek the Comforter.

Just so that you understand that the Comforter is for you, you already called on Him and He already lifted you. The Comforter was there when you lost that baby, when you lost that court case, when you lost that job, when your husband cheated, when you cheated, when you changed, when your family abandoned you, when you were financially challenged, when you were spiritually broken, and all the other things that encumbers you.

I left you a Comforter, so you should access your Comforter for your distress rather than those things that cause you to sin.

I expect you to access the Holy Spirit.

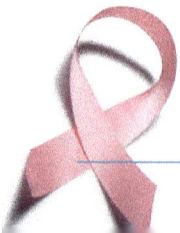

Romans 8:26-27 (NIV) [26] In the same way, the Spirit helps us in our weakness. We do not know what we ought to pray for, but the Spirit himself intercedes for us through wordless groans. [27] And He who searches our hearts knows the mind of the Spirit, because the Spirit intercedes for God's people in accordance with the will of God.

I have given you an intercessor.

Oh the Holy Spirit! What a gift! When you do not know what to pray for or what to do, you have the Holy Spirit. The main complaint is that you do not know when the Holy Spirit is talking to you. I have a distinct voice, so likewise so does the Holy Spirit. Keep listening. You are listening for My words and My wisdom. What would I say to you in your situation? What does My word say about your situation? Who have I sent to you do offer wise counsel and information? Are you focused on what I am saying to you?

One step toward hearing is being still. A second step for hearing is being quiet. Another important part is clearing your mind from doubt and fear and sabotage. The next step is to remember that My voice is one of love, which cancels your self-hatred and personal demise.

I gave you someone who knows My will and My ways who does not second guess Me or My message, who does not get sidetracked by the world and its trappings, someone who can focus on Me, and who can follow My directions faithfully and without questions.

I have made provisions for My will to be completed. Access your intercessor with faith, hope and love.

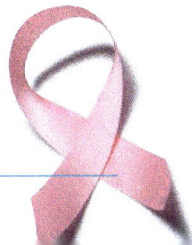

Psalm 115:12a (NIV) [12] The LORD remembers us and will bless us: He will bless his people Israel; he will bless the house of Aaron,

I bless you.

I bless you. I bless you like I blessed Isaac, Ishmael, Noah, David, Naomi, Ruth, Esther, Joseph, Job, Matthew, Mark, Luke, John, Mary, Elizabeth, Paul, Nathan, Lazarus, and other unnamed persons.

I bless you, even when you don't think that I have. I know that you don't like to struggle. Your struggles and its outcomes function as your testimony; part of your life story.

When you share your testimony with others, they are reassured that I am the real God—the God of their prayers and yours.

I bless you so that you can bless others. I bless you so that you can bless others. You are not the decision maker about who I bless with the testimony I provide!

I know that some of your testimony is embarrassing but you are not authorized to edit My results. I am the Author of that testimony. It is designed to save someone else or to redeem someone else. Any omissions or edits may cause the person to question what they need to do to get that testimony and how they can get My help. Their situation is not too hard for Me. I am going to insure that they have access to Me.

I bless you!

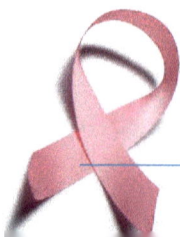

Exodus 14:14 (NIV) [14] The LORD will fight for you; you need only to be still."

I fight your battles.

And I do not need your help, support or consent. I know that being still is a challenge, but I am still God. I am not sure what else I need to say because that is the fact and nothing more is necessary.

We also define battle differently. What you label as a battle is not what I label a battle. The other important part of this is that I have all outcomes planned; even those non-battles.

When your boss is trying to terminate you, I handle that. When your children are trying to sabotage you and themselves, I handle them. When you and your husband wanted to divorce but you had a change of heart and some other significant changes happened, that was Me. When you were in surgery and there was an equipment malfunction, you survived because I was there and I kept you alive.

I give both a voice and a platform after these battles. These battles and the subsequent victories are to bring Me glory and honor and worship and praise. I love you and I fight your battles. I choose you to fight for because I need to trust you to share My work with all others.

I prepare you for the battles which I fight!

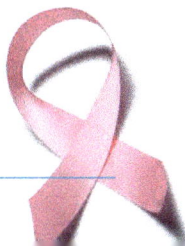

Ephesians 6:10-18 (NIV) [10] Finally, be strong in the Lord and in His mighty power. [11] Put on the full armor of God, so that you can take your stand against the devil's schemes. [12] For our struggle is not against flesh and blood, but against the rulers, against the authorities, against the powers of this dark world and against the spiritual forces of evil in the heavenly realms. [13] Therefore put on the full armor of God, so that when the day of evil comes, you may be able to stand your ground, and after you have done everything, to stand.

I provide protection.

I provide protection for all of My disciples, soldiers, warriors, and other persons I have called. My full armor is comprehensive. You make Me protect you without all of the pieces.

Why do you wear half of the armor which I so freely provide? That armor is in place to facilitate victory over the struggle you consistently request relief from.

There's the helmet of salvation. You wear that part-time. The fact that you wear the armor part-time leaves you open and vulnerable to the devil's schemes. You are the reason that you are a target.

The belt of truth, the breast plate of righteousness, feet fitted with readiness, shield of faith, helmet of salvation, and the sword of the Spirit. These six pieces of My comprehensive armor are essential, but you refuse some of the pieces of My armor randomly. I created the pieces to work together as a unit. The pieces are not really stand alone. Use all of them at the same time. Please and Thank You.

I provide your protection; that very high hedge around you!

Put on the armor! Now! Quit taking it off!

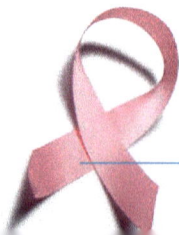

Philippians 4:7 (NIV) [7] And the peace of God, which transcends all understanding, will guard your hearts and your minds in Christ Jesus.

I provide your peace.

I try not to get frustrated or angry with you but you make it really hard. Stop seeking peace in other places! I am the Source of your peace. Your peace does not come from the mall, your friends, your marriage or significant other, a bottle, pills, drugs, or anything else. Those very items, events, and people tend to cause you additional unrest.

When you need peace, I am your Source. Without Me, you cannot experience true peace. Stop hoping that something can take My place or do My job. And then after the shabby substitute fails you, you are back to praying to Me, hoping I move on your schedule.

I am your peace! I do not need your help, or any other assistance. Your substitute is not even close to helping your situation.

I am your peace! Quite the provider, I might add. I quiet your thoughts, your worries. I help you sleep at night when you go to bed worried and scared, scarred from your life and circumstances. I am your peace!

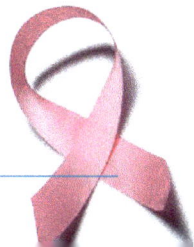

1 Peter 5:7 (NIV) [7] Cast all your anxiety on Him because He cares for you.

I receive your anxieties.

I accept your anxieties! I really do. You have anxieties because your faith is weak and challenged. I am the only one willing to take your anxieties on so that you can give up and return to a strong faith.

I will take those anxieties because they lead to worry and angst and fear and burdens. These take you away from Me, and keeps you from praising, worshipping and praying.

Although I remind you regularly to stop keeping those anxieties to yourself or even letting them become anxieties, you do so anyway. Then I still take them.

I care about you! I love you! I keep you! I keep you whole! I want your anxieties so that I can have you whole and to Myself. When you are anxious, I am forced to share. I do not share. I am a jealous God. I will not share you with your anxieties and worries and fears. I did not create you like that or to do that.

You gain nothing by holding on to them. Give them to Me—without reservation and unapologetically.

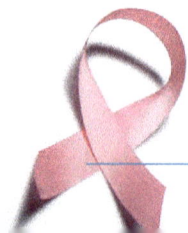

John 16:33 (NIV) [33] "I have told you these things, so that in Me you may have peace. In this world you will have trouble. But take heart! I have overcome the world."

I did not give you anything that I cannot handle.

I have shown you through My Son, Jesus Christ, that I can overcome the entire world. Jesus shares the preceding scriptures so that you will have an understanding, although you often forget what you have been taught or what you have been given access to. I have given you the answers to many questions, even those which are never asked.

Jesus offers peace in a life which promises trouble. Jesus then encourages you to take heart—remain focused! I have assigned you to do things based on the gifts I have given to you for the people which I have assigned to you. I have prepared you for **all** that comes in your direction. Those events, persons and incidents are specifically designed for your attention, education and your opportunity to grow.

All of that considers that I have charge over your situation—which I do. Everywhere you are and everything that happens to you is under My control.

So complete My assignments and tasks and give to My people as I have gifted you to do so. I have prepared your path for My glory and My praise. So your path will be troubled and complicated but I will supply you with what you need to carry out My will.

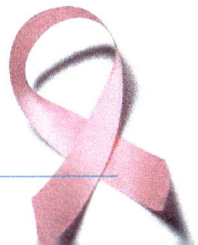

Philippians 4:6 (NIV) [6] Do not be anxious about anything, but in every situation, by prayer and petition, with thanksgiving, present your requests to God.

I am listening to you. I hear you each and every time you pray.

I have told you several times, in several ways that your anxiety prevents you from hearing Me. Your misplaced anxiety keeps your path cluttered and your thoughts clouded.

I am listening to you—that should stop some of your anxiety. What are you anxious about anyway? I feed you. I clothe you. I employ you. I create opportunities for you to be successful. I put you in front of people that I need you to serve and those I need to serve you.

I am listening to You! I am concerned about you. I am considerate of you. I think about you. I plan for you. I clean up after you and the mess you create.

I am attentive to you and your prayers and your prayer requests. I am paying attention to you! Stop asking Me if I can hear you! Prayer is Our conversation. There are prayers which are not in My will which I will deny. I think that you need to remember that I am God. My plans have never failed. I am going to deliver the best outcome for all that are affected. Relax in My Word and My peace.

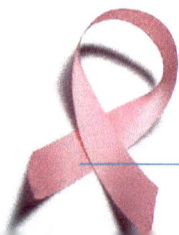

Isaiah 26:2 (NIV) ³ You will keep in perfect peace those whose minds are steadfast, because they trust in you.

You should trust Me.

I will keep you in perfect peace if you trust Me. And only Me! That is Our real issue. You don't actually trust Me—at least not all of the time. You selectively trust Me. You don't want Me to trust you selectively, so why do you trust Me selectively? You don't have a good answer; you don't even have any good evidence that supports your behavior.

You need peace right now more than ever! Your health and heart and mind and soul need My peace right now. You are thirsty for answers and seeking answers. You are challenged by your current condition. You need to learn to trust Me. Your future depends on you trusting Me—unconditionally. Let Us reflect on the areas of your life which still causes you awe and wonder. I saved your life. . . .several times actually. I revealed the family "secrets" to you so that you could intervene. When I saved your child's life, I allowed you to be a vessel to do that work. I have financed your life when you were not supposed to be able to afford it or have the credit worthiness to do so either. You should trust Me. I deserve your trust and should not have to continue to prove My trustworthiness to you.

Trust.

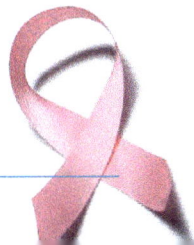

Hebrews 11:6 (NIV) [6] And without faith it is impossible to please God, because anyone who comes to him must believe that he exists and that he rewards those who earnestly seek him.

I want you to prove Me right.

Faith in Me is critical for Our relationship to be real. Our relationship is based on what We do for each other, including how We communicate with each other, how We interact with each other, and how We respond to each other.

I am God. I am everybody's God and I alone will be praised. If you have faith in the God who created you and gives you life daily and supply your needs to an unbelievable proportion of what you have requested, and so much more than what you needed. Faith is required because I have the full picture of what is going to happen next.

If you do not believe, then why do you pray? Why do you believe part-time? Why do you selectively believe in Me and what you ask Me for? Do you think that I deserve your trust? Do I deserve your faith? Have I done anything that causes you to have no or limited faith in Me or that causes you to question or second-guess Me, My plans and My process?

If you are faithful to Me, then you will prove that I am the God you invited into your heart and as the Leader of your life. Prove Me right through your unwavering faith.

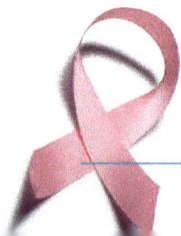

Philippians 4:13 (NIV) [13] I can do all this through Him who gives me strength.

I equip you to do everything I have given you.

Have you been really paying attention to Me? I do not give you anything to do or to become that you do not already have the tools to be successful! With this fact in mind, why are you in doubt? I know that you doubt because of your questions and your behavior! You ask Me questions which exude doubt. You completely quit right before I can deliver the best part: the results. I cannot understand why you let some of the most minor situations cause your faith to waiver.

Your lack of faith communicates your distrust for Me. Why is that? What do you disbelieve in My plan? Why do you lack confidence in yourself? Didn't you grow when you were awarded that promotion? Didn't your faith grow when you child recovered from that illness? Didn't you become more faithful when I answered your prayers for your family?

Yes, I am going to challenge you. I challenged everyone before you: Jacob, Noah, Boaz, Ananias, Timothy, and everyone else! I will challenge everyone after you as well. I challenge you not to prove who you are to Me, but to prove who you are and what you actually capable to yourself. This is how I show you who you are.

Philippians 2:14-16 (NIV) [14] Do everything without grumbling or arguing, [15] so that you may become blameless and pure, "children of God without fault in a warped and crooked generation." Then you will shine among them like stars in the sky [16] as you hold firmly to the word of life. And then I will be able to boast on the day of Christ that I did not run or labor in vain.

I am building your character for My next assignment.

You can always use more character and more confidence for what you consider difficult. What you forget is that others are watching your behavior to determine whether I can be their God.

Because I am constantly proving to you who you are, I am also preparing you for your next assignment. I am in need of your focus to complete this task as well as the next tasks.

If I am building you, your character and your tenacity, then you need to recognize that I am invested in you and how you will function in My will.

I created you to function within My will. You exist to move My will forward. You cannot continue to try to quit or take a break. My will has a timing that has to move on time. You cannot delay My will and I do not like the idea that you may get distracted from My plan. As a part of that character, I will move and remove anyone and anything that distracts you from My will and My plan. My will be done.

You will be challenged because of Me. You need to stay focused on Me. Your next assignment is bigger and more important than the ones before.

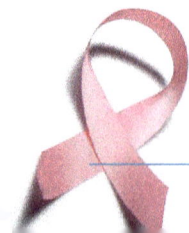

Philippians 2:17-18 (NIV) [17] But even if I am being poured out like a drink offering on the sacrifice and service coming from your faith, I am glad and rejoice with all of you. [18] So you too should be glad and rejoice with me.

I want you to find reasons and ways to rejoice.

You are My child! I know you! I know that your outlook on life sometimes slips from outstanding to bleak. One incident, one wrong word, one lost job, one divorce, or affair, can move you from blissful to depressed.

Joy does not work like this. Joy exists through and survives the issue, which in the grand scheme is minimal and does not interrupt My will. When several events and results combine to become your testimony, that isolated incident is part of a larger picture and is not as debilitating as it was when you initially encountered it.

Find reasons to be joyful. There's joy in your life. Pick through all of it to find the joy which I have provided for you. Joy keeps you totally focused on Me. Find or learn ways to rejoice. Find ways to see Me and My hands in your life, especially in these issues and incidents.

Everything you endure has a purpose. Please look for joy so that you can spread that joy around to others, because I assigned them to you.

Joy is part of life—the life that I provide and the one to come.

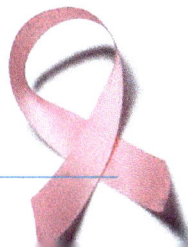

Philippians 1:27-28 (NIV) [27] Whatever happens, conduct yourselves in a manner worthy of the gospel of Christ. Then, whether I come and see you or only hear about you in my absence, I will know that you stand firm in the one Spirit, striving together as one for the faith of the gospel [28] without being frightened in any way by those who oppose you. This is a sign to them that they will be destroyed, but that you will be saved—and that by God.

I want others to see My hand in your life.

You should want others to see My hand in your life. You should want Me to get credit for My work in your life. My plans and blessings are miraculous and awesome and breath taking. I want you to recognize My work, My hand in your life, so that you can recognize My definition of your worth. My hand loves you and cares for you and keeps you whole and healthy and gifts you and shows you My way.

My hand forgives you, gives you the ability to love, and the love supply, which I replenish all of the time.

My hand teaches love, commands that you love others, and demonstrates the love I expect for you to shower on others. Regardless of your definition of their worth. I placed you in a position to love others, not to decide whether they deserve your love. The evidence of My hand is your unconditional love to others.

Your life is not perfect. Your life is waiting on My hand, the evidence of My presence. Sometimes you need to be reminded. Others need to see My hand all of the time.

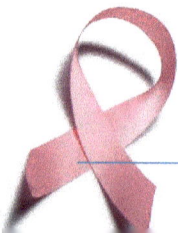

Philippians 2:1-4 (NIV) Therefore if you have any encouragement from being united with Christ, if any comfort from His love, if any common sharing in the Spirit, if any tenderness and compassion, [2] then make my joy complete by being like-minded, having the same love, being one in spirit and of one mind. [3] Do nothing out of selfish ambition or vain conceit. Rather, in humility value others above yourselves, [4] not looking to your own interests but each of you to the interests of the others.

I equipped and designed you to help others.

As your Creator, I designed you for helping others. I did that on purpose. You helping others benefits Me and the both of you. Why do you have to help others?

Because I said so and someone else helped you. I have assigned someone to you to help you. I am committed to you so that you can serve others as I have commanded.

I have gifted each of you with each other and talents which allow and equip you to support each other. Through this support and service, you are able to demonstrate the love that I command of you.

Why are you against helping others? Why are you avoiding helping others? Does it harm you to help others? Do you understand that when you help others, the person(s) you help experience Me? Do you know that you are serving Me when you help others?

Just based on those questions, do you think I want something that is unfair of you? Helping is not a punishment. Helping is a an act of obedience to Me. Helping others is praise and worship to Me.

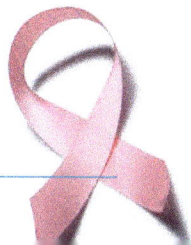

Ephesians 4:26-27 (NIV) [26] "In your anger do not sin": Do not let the sun go down while you are still angry, [27] and do not give the devil a foothold.

I want you to channel your anger to Me and My work.

Anger is useful when you use that anger to accomplish a goal or to help someone in need or when you overcome your fears about something. Anger could be good to motivate you to do the next thing. Anger could be used to damage everything in your path. Anger can cause issues and rifts and discord and damage, some of which is irreparable. Your anger stops progress within yourself and others. Your anger causes others to misunderstand good logic. In your anger, do not sin. Yet, you do sin anyway. You sin based on some weird circumstances and situations. You sin in ways which require extensive forgiveness and healing. When your anger causes you this much work, you need to reconsider whether that anger is worth it.

I want that anger to become productive for your life. The energy required for maintaining anger could be used to complete that project that you started last year or that book you are scared to write or to return to school. Anger is useful to overcome your fear and anxiety. Share your anger with Me so I can help you channel it effectively.

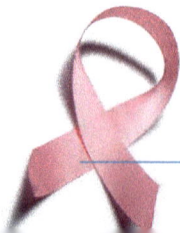

James 1:19-20 (NIV) [19] My dear brothers and sisters, take note of this: Everyone should be quick to listen, slow to speak and slow to become angry, [20] because human anger does not produce the righteousness that God desires.

I do not want you so angry that you forget your purpose.

There are angry people all around you, including you. That anger and your consumption with it. Oh yes, you are concerned with anger and it's built on many different situations and involves many people, because you have never forgiven them for all that they have done, nor have you forgiven yourself. You are so angry that you consistently reject love, forgiveness and relationships. Sometimes you are angry with Me. This is a real issue.

I can just love you through your anger. I have not been able to remove that anger because you hold onto it tighter than you can ever hold onto Me. You have convinced yourself that this is the only way to survive: to keep that anger alive because if you have to heal, I am your healer and you would have to surrender … to Me.

Your anger interrupts your purpose, the purpose I have given you, I am so disappointed that we are having this dilemma. Your anger is supposed to propel you to the excellence I have prepared you for and for that which I have prepared for you. Your anger was designed to get your attention so that you could return to Me, not resort to the pitiful revenge that you feel will satisfy and solution your anger.

Surrender your anger to Me. Let it go.

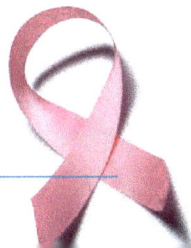

Proverbs 12:25 (NIV) [25] Anxiety weighs down the heart, but a kind word cheers it up.

I am in control. There's no need to be anxious.

Why do I have to remind you that I am in control? I have the total view of your situation, every aspect: emotional, financial, spiritual, and physical. I am in total control of the entirety of your being and all of it's details.

Remember when you thought you were going to lose your child but you didn't? You trusted Me more then than you do now.

I am the Lord, your God, who brought your family across the desert, made wet land dry for their escape, healed your land which I provided, and loved you even when you do not listen or obey.

I know that you are sick and in need of healing. I know that you are uncomfortable with your job. I know that you want more money and more time and just more. I know that you want to have more exposure for your talents and more financial security. I know that you are concerned about your children.

I know that you are anxious about the issues that you have. I am right here. I have not left you. I have not stopped saving you from yourself. I am in control. Stop trying to do My job.

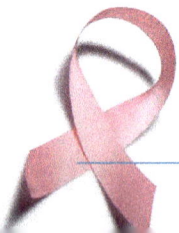

Philippians 4:6 (NIV) [6] Do not be anxious about anything, but in every situation, by prayer and petition, with thanksgiving, present your requests to God.

I want to hear everything you have to say. Always.

I am our God—Your Father. I created you. I planned you and I planned a life for you. I give you gifts and talents. I give you what you need and some of the desires of your heart. I am your Source of your healing, strength, and love.

I am your sounding board—I am listening to your prayers. I am your God. I am listening to you. I hear you. I am paying attention to you. You are not alone. You are not by yourself.

I know you have questions. I know that you want My answers. I know you don't understand My methods or My techniques but I am God and God alone. I am not always going to fix what you want fixed immediately and sometimes not at all; at least not the way you requested it.

I am going to answer you and grant you what you need for My will to be done. I consider My will the best avenue for all that you are and what you need. I hope that you come to that same conclusion soon.

Just because you don't get the answer that you want, when you want it and how you want it, does not mean that My ears are closed.

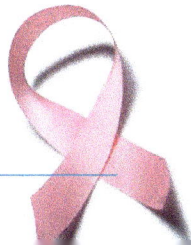

Hebrews 4:12 (NIV) [12] For the word of God is alive and active. Sharper than any double-edged sword, it penetrates even to dividing soul and spirit, joints and marrow; it judges the thoughts and attitudes of the heart.

I am purifying your heart.

I can actually identify all of the events, incidents, and people who have caused negative changes in your heart. From your first love to your divorce, from your losing your job to losing your children, from being evicted to having your car repossessed, I know the exact time your heart hardened; every time it hardened.

I teach lessons during these times. I show you who I really am during the worst parts of your lives and during those times when life seems at its worst.

I want your heart to return to its purest form because a pure heart will see Me without conditions or with questionable motives. Your heart is driven by motives. Your verbal responses are a result of your heart's condition. If I can return your heart to the original state of purity so that I can offer it to others, so that you can really serve Me with all your heart, then I would. Right now you are only serving Me with about 37% of your heart. 37% is quite far from 100%, the definition of whole.

I think you will like yourself better and you will definitely understand what I know about you if your heart was closer to pure.

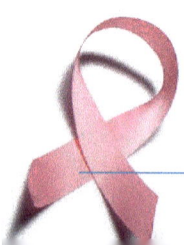

Hebrews 11:1 (NIV) [1] Now faith is confidence in what we hope for and assurance about what we do not see.

I want you to have better, stronger faith. Unwavering.

You place Me in a box which does not afford you the opportunity to understand the extent of My will. You let the world separate us because they challenge you on who I am and what I do but mostly what they don't thing I can or will do.

When do you simply believe and not question Me? What do I have to do to earn your faith? I already provide you breath to breathe. I bless you with the use of your limbs and all other organs. I bless you with wisdom, knowledge, and intellect daily. I bless you with employment with a salary and healthcare benefits. I bless you with a marriage and a children. I bless you with gifts and talents so that you can make My will happen. I gave you compassion and love and empathy to help others.

I send others to you who I can trust to serve and bless you based on My will and what you request in prayer.

Your faith is required for you to grow. If you do not have faith in Me, why should I listen to you or answer you or pay attention to you? I require faith in Me. I need to trust you.

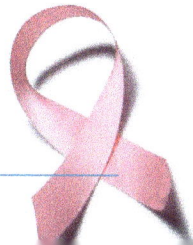

Titus 2:1, 3-5 (NIV) [1] You, however, must teach what is appropriate to sound doctrine. [3] Likewise, teach the older women to be reverent in the way they live, not to be slanderers or addicted to much wine, but to teach what is good. [4] Then they can urge the younger women to love their husbands and children, [5] to be self-controlled and pure, to be busy at home, to be kind, and to be subject to their husbands, so that no one will malign the word of God.

I expect you to teach and share your testimony.

I gifted you with a gift and a talent. Those gifts and talents are to be shared with others. One of our major issues is cooperation with one another. This cooperative arrangement is what propels every continent forward. I am working on all of you working together for what the kingdom needs. I am committed to you using your gifts. I am your God and God alone. I am gifting new teachers daily, hourly even, but I need you to actually teach. You also need to share your testimony but you don't want to because you are embarrassed and ashamed, but I gave you that testimony to share with those I have sent who need it.

Your testimony helps you witness to others about Christ. Your testimony is your message and that message is divinely tailored for your audience. This testimony will need to be honest and transparent. You need to be authentic when you share your testimony. I need you to remember that I am the Author of that testimony—I gave you what I need you to share. Do not edit or change or alter or omit My testimony.

Teach and share. Non-negotiable. Not optional.

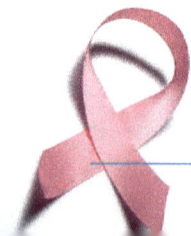

2 Timothy 2:15 (NIV) [15] Do your best to present yourself to God as one approved, a worker who does not need to be ashamed and who correctly handles the word of truth.

I expect you to study.

I am God. You are not. Jesus is the closest being to Me and even He studies. He studied, prayed, fasted, taught and performed miracles, amongst the other wonders.

I expect you to study. Read. Study. Read. Meditate. Read. Pray. Read. Share. Read. Ask questions. Read. Meditate. Read. Put My word into practice. Everyday. All Day. Without excuse.

Non-Christians are prepared to challenge you. If they can challenge you, then they can change you. You need to be prepared with the scripture text and what it means. If you don't want to be challenged, then STUDY! My word does not come to unprepared hearts and minds. In order to be able to recall My words in your time of need, you have to study, memorize and live.

I expect you to study because I will need you to use what I have written and spoken. I need you available to work. In order to work, you have to train. All activities require training. The Bible is not different—you need to read and know the related and supporting scriptures. When you are approached by someone who says that I am not real, what are you going to say?

Study.

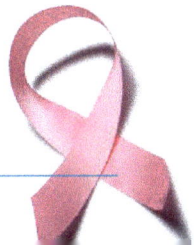

Romans 12:10-11, 13 (NIV) [10] Be devoted to one another in love. Honor one another above yourselves. [11] Never be lacking in zeal, but keep your spiritual fervor, serving the Lord. [13] Share with the Lord's people who are in need. Practice hospitality.

I expect you to continue or start to serve others.

Who did I send to serve you? Do you remember who introduced Me to you? I do. I remember every person who helped lead you to Me. I know every usher, greeter, Sunday school teacher, Bible study lesson and leader. I remember every question you asked, every comment you offered, every praise, every workshop, and every prayer.

I remember everyone that I exposed you to so that you would come to Me. I have sent believers and non-believers food, projects, events, victories, tragedies, employment and unemployment.

I need you to be obedient to the Holy Spirit when I send people who are out of relationship with Me, so that you can minister to them about Me. I am going to position you in place where people have questions, need guidance and are hurting. I need you to help them through these areas with tools you have which are designed to help others whom I send to you.

Ask others do they have a relationship with Me. With Jesus Christ. Then invite them to church with you, then pray about what to do next. Keep your heart focused on Me. I will keep you in perfect peace.

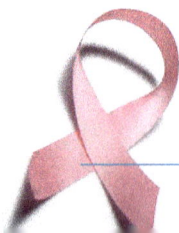

Romans 12:14, 16-18 (NIV) [14] Bless those who persecute you; bless and do not curse. [16] Live in harmony with one another. Do not be proud, but be willing to associate with people of low position. Do not be conceited. [17] Do not repay anyone evil for evil. Be careful to do what is right in the eyes of everyone. [18] If it is possible, as far as it depends on you, live at peace with everyone.

I expect you to help those around you to reconcile.

I am really intense about forgiveness. I have made several statements about forgiveness. You still remain disobedient about forgiveness. You are selectively forgiving and selectively obedient. My will be done, which includes your forgiveness and teaching others to do so as well. I am concerned that you think that it's not important to Me. I am not going to listen to your pitiful prayers if you do not forgive others. You are not too good to forgive others. I know that you are hurting. I am your healer. I take care of what others do to you.

Now you have to forgive through the toughest of times for you to be able to support reconciliation. First of all, please do not negate the reconciliation even if you cannot support it. Secondly, I need you to reunite so that the devil is omitted. Separation gives the devil a foothold. Reconciliation makes the unit stronger. I need stronger units, so reconciliation is required.

I need you to teach, foster, and perpetuate reconciliation. Be a problem solver. The solution. Be the solution! Hold them accountable for the solution and its outcome.

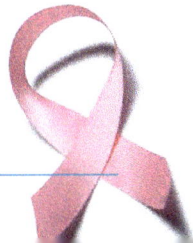

Romans 12:12 (NIV) [12] Be joyful in hope, patient in affliction, faithful in prayer.

I want you to have a great attitude.

That verse reads 'patient in affliction' because I use you and your trials to increase the faith of yourself and others in My kingdom. I further use those afflictions to show the world who I am and what I am capable of doing. Keep focused on Me and not the affliction. The affliction will hurt but the outcome will minimize, and possibly, erase the pain. The next assignment is based on this assignment.

I want you to understand that you were chosen for your assignment. While you may never totally know, you were chosen and I know that you want your life to be different, you still know that I am God and I am in charge and in control. I am growing you up for excellence according to My definition. Your growth and development is critical for My plans. I am clear that we are not on the same page about how I orchestrate My plans. I do want you to understand that because I have the entire plan, I do not honor some of your requests. Some of your requests would sabotage My plan completely, because they are in complete contradiction to what I need to have in the works.

I need you to smile and be joyful.

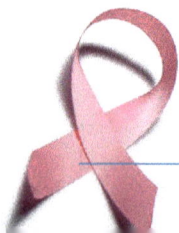

Ephesians 2:8 (NIV) [8] For it is by grace you have been saved, through faith—and this is not from yourselves, it is the gift of God

You are My best work.

When I put the plans of the world in motion, I designed you, then at the proper time, I created you. You are My best work. Yes, you are. I planned you for the work that you would do. You are My best work for the assignment that you have. I am amazed that you continue to doubt your abilities and further more you doubt My abilities to assign you to do something that I have equipped you to do.

I know that you are worried and scared about your assignment and the outcome but I really mean for you to understand your best abilities.

Stop doubting. Stop questioning. Stop debating. Stop disbelieving. Stop arguing. Stop stressing. Stop being confused. Stop analyzing. Stop whining. Stop complaining.

You are My best work. Sometimes, however, you do not show up to work and when you do show up, you are not at your best. I get some sloppy work from you. You are lazy and you complain like no one I have ever created.

Please stop doubting the abilities which I have given you. I am God. I know what I am doing. Trust.

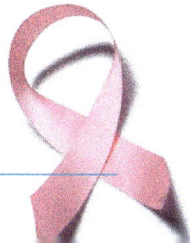

Isaiah 41:10 (NIV) [10] So do not fear, for I am with you; do not be dismayed, for I am your God. I will strengthen you and help you; I will uphold you with my righteous right hand.

I am your God.

You need to understand what that means. I am your God. That means that I am your Source—for everything. I need to remind you that I am your God, your Creator, your Source because you try to replace Me with liquor, drugs, degrees, sex, shopping, or whatever else you 'go-to' first before Me.

I do not come behind those details. I am FIRST. I am not sure why I need to keep reminding you of that. It's annoying to tell you who I am and to remind you of what I do.

I am your God means I keep your employed. I keep you financially afloat. I keep your kids in school. I reunited your family. I answer your prayers. I meet your needs. I keep the enemy away from you. I watch over you, especially when you try to sabotage yourself with certain activities. I listen to you and I make you whole.

I am your God. I have given you gifts that you did not expect. I have blessed you with knowledge and wisdom. I answer your prayers. I provide for you so that you can do My will.

I am your God.

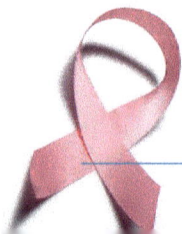

2 Corinthians 12:10 (NIV) [10] That is why, for Christ's sake, I delight in weaknesses, in insults, in hardships, in persecutions, in difficulties. For when I am weak, then I am strong.

I am at My best in your life—right now.

As I define best, I am doing around you what I need for your good and My will. Paul shares with you that he boasts in his weakness because of Christ's grace and power. This is hard for most of you. You are not able to tell people when you are weak or suffering or in hardship or having difficulties because you are proud or embarrassed or ashamed or all of the above.

There are some things that I have to demonstrate to the world and I use you to demonstrate these messages.

Now, when I bless you after these difficulties, you are not embarrassed, or ashamed or upset. When people comment on your blessings, you manage to share the blessing story but not the 'before' story. I bless you for My glory, but I do not always get that glory and praise.

I am more concerned about how others see Me in your weakness. The world expects for you to fail in your weakness, but your faith in Me says otherwise. The world wants to know and I expect you to tell them that you are surviving this situation because I am sustaining you.

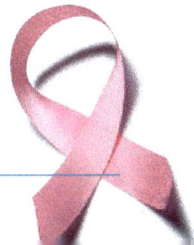

1 Corinthians 13 (MSG) [13] But for right now, until that completeness, we have three things to do to lead us toward that consummation: Trust steadily in God, hope unswervingly, love extravagantly. And the best of the three is love.

You are love—act like it. All the time!

Love is a verb. I love you in action. My love for you has been demonstrated through your salvation, your life and its blessings.

I designed you to love. I love you. I give you love to give away. You are to walk in love and all that goes with it. No envy. No strife. No jealousy. No anger. When you are having a hard time loving, come talk to Me. First of all, you are not the supplier or replenisher of your love or your ability to love. You love like you are going to run out. I supply your love and I give you the ability to love. I am your definition of love. I have shown you how to love. I have shown you how to love. I have told you who to love: everyone!

Love is not selective. You cannot pick who to love because of whatever reason. I said love your neighbor as yourself but the reason that you don't love everyone is because you also selectively love yourself. You are supposed to love yourself as well.

This is not optional—love is required. Be love. Act like love, even if you don't feel like it. Love is essential to all that I do and all that I am. Love created you! There are no breaks from love.

Love is a full-time activity.

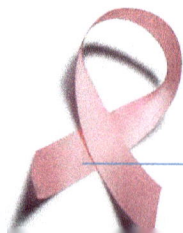

Matthew 18:19-20 (NIV) [19] "Again, truly I tell you that if two of you on earth agree about anything they ask for, it will be done for them by My Father in heaven. [20] For where two or three gather in My name, there am I with them."

This is a perfect time to gather with others and pray.

Everyday there is a reason to pray. Crime. Theft. Abductions. Legal injustice. Elections. Illness. Financial unrest. Civil unrest. Education. Health care. Leadership. Authority. Hate. Hatred. Government. Lack of democracy. Hunger. Homelessness. Unemployment. Broken marriages. Broken families. People who are hurting. People who are grieving. People who are in prison unjustly. People who don't know Me.

Gather with others who you know and do not know to pray or how to pray. I know that everyone has some issues that they need to share with Me for themselves or on behalf of others. Your prayers fall on My attentive ears and My willing heart.

Gathering is My idea for communing and love and cohesiveness. When you pray, I am listening. When you pray with others, then you have My undivided attention and My attention to your requests heightens.

When you are in agreement and not in conflict, I am glorified. That's what matters most.

Your unity brings glory to My name.

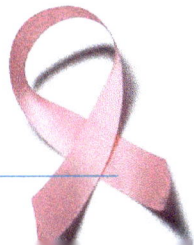

2 Timothy 3:16-17 (NIV) [16] All Scripture is God-breathed and is useful for teaching, rebuking, correcting and training in righteousness, [17] so that the servant of God may be thoroughly equipped for every good work.

I built you an Instruction Manual. Use it.

I put together an Instruction Manual, better known as the Bible. I have spoken through more than 200 people to create that Manual. Those stories and instructions and words of wisdom and historical encounters are useful for your daily life. These pages are comprehensive for your life. I have given you instructions for situations when you need it. I have given you words of advice and wisdom. I have given you the stories of some great characters who have first-hand knowledge of My love, direction, discipline, and power.

This Manual needs to be the first Source after Me. Right now it is accessed on a haphazard basis. You just read it on occasion, rather than daily and all of it. The answers to some of your issues are in writing and completely accessible to you, but you do not.

I insist that you use the Instruction Manual because I provided it. I built the Manual over many years with many people. You need it and I developed it because I love you and I provide for you. This is one such major provision.

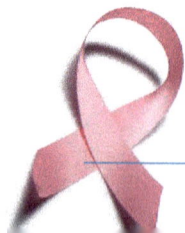

Matthew 21:22 (NIV) [22] If you believe, you will receive whatever you ask for in prayer."

I am testing your belief.

I have asked you to believe, because I see that doubt that you harbor and rehearse and use regularly. You hold that doubt tightly, but I am not sure why. Your belief should have more power than your doubt, but your belief is weak against your doubt. The problem is that you have plenty reasons to believe.

If you don't believe in what you are asking, then why should I be the One who changes your mind? I am not going to convince you to believe in Me or your requests.

For the last time, either believe or quit asking. Belief means that you ask and not question when or how or for what reason. Belief means that you ask without doubt of the outcome. Belief means that you ask with some certainty that you will be granted your request.

I need you to quit wavering between belief and disbelief. That wavering attitude is the problem I have with you. Faith cannot waiver. Faith in Me should be constant.

I am going to test you—absolutely. You need to focus on Me and My word.

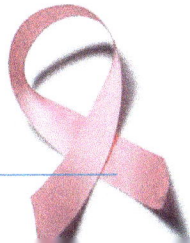

Psalm 37:4 (NIV) [4] Take delight in the LORD, and He will give you the desires of your heart.

Take delight in Me, I will give you the desires of your heart.

Take delight in me, I will give you the desires of your heart—according to My will. What does delight in Me look like? Prayer, especially when you do not feel like it and when you do not feel the need to pray. Repenting because of your sins and your shortcomings. Helping those that I place in your path. Using your gifts and talents at the proper time; without complaint and humbly.

Following My directions, especially when they are difficult and when you are the only one following the directions. Staying away from temptation, especially when I provide an escape. Being kind and compassionate to one another, especially after someone has harmed you. Forgive others who harm you, especially when you don't want to. Praise Me in spirit and in truth, even when you do not want to praise Me, regardless of the reason.

Share Me with others, even though you are shy and scared. Serve me with all that you are and all that you are not. Love Me with all your heart and your mind and your soul. Delight means that you share Me. Glorify Me. Praise Me. Take delight in Me.

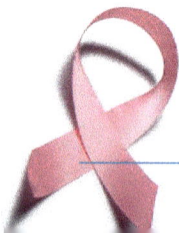

Genesis 2:7 (NIV) [7] Then the LORD God formed a man from the dust of the ground and breathed into his nostrils the breath of life, and the man became a living being.

I do everything for you.

When I breathed air into your lungs, I decided to start the plans I have for you. This act is by far the first step for the rest of your life. I have been breathing into your lungs daily since your inception. And I will continue to breathe into your lungs until your work is complete. I am the deciding factor on the definition of completion.

I breathe for you. I eat for you and I digest for you. I inhale for you. I exhale for you. I move fluids around in your body so that you have just the right amount of insulin and waste. I regulate your eye sight and your hearing. I regulate the percentage of your brain usage.

I help you to love and for others to love you. I put people in your path and put you in the path of others for the purpose of My will. I share ideas and thoughts with you for the advancement of My kingdom through the work of your hands and the creativity of your mind and the freedom of your spirit and the openness of your heart.

I do all of that for you. I made you in My image.

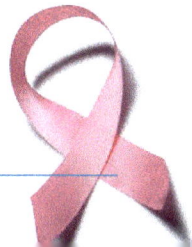

Galatians 5:22-23 (NIV) [22] But the fruit of the Spirit is love, joy, peace, forbearance, kindness, goodness, faithfulness, [23] gentleness and self-control. Against such things there is no law.

I have given you some characteristics that I want you to emphasize.

I need the fruit of the Spirit to be dominant in your life and your daily and regular interactions with others. This is how others will know that you belong to Me. Love. Joy. Forbearance. Kindness. Goodness. Faithfulness. Gentleness. Self-control. While there are nine separate parts, be reminded that the Fruit is one whole element. I need you to work on all of the nine details. There are harder elements than others to perfect and exhibit. For those which are harder, please submit those to Me for My guidance and assistance. Each detail is critical. One hinges on the next. They all need to be present. They have to co-exist. They complement each other.

Make no excuses about your effort toward the elements. You are equipped to make it happen. Remember to share the Fruit—they are best when shared. Love others, Me and yourself at all times, under all circumstances, for all reasons, and because I loved you first and unconditionally. Be joyful because I give it to you, no matter what. Be peace and peaceful because I give you that. Forbearance through the perceived difficulties. Be kind to all because they seek you for kindness. Goodness is your measure toward righteousness—did you do the right thing? Faithfulness to Me is required—not a part-time faith, rather a full-time, never quitting, never tiring, never failing faith. Gentleness means to treat My people, all of them, with a subtle firmness which leaves them whole and better than they arrived. Self-control restricts your responses and activities; means saying no and not sharing the fullness of your most authentic feelings.

I need all of them immediately, available to those I send in your service.

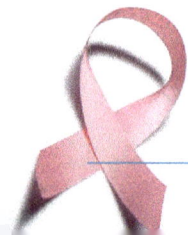

Matthew 28:19-20 (NIV) [19] Therefore go and make disciples of all nations, baptizing them in the name of the Father and of the Son and of the Holy Spirit, [20] and teaching them to obey everything I have commanded you. And surely I am with you always, to the very end of the age."

Are you sharing Me with others?

Go ye therefore and make disciples of all nations! Teaching and baptizing them. Are you doing what I commanded you to do? Are you sharing Me with others?

Someone shared Me with you, obediently and reverently. Someone I sent to you to share Me with you who attempted to explain Me and worship Me and praise Me. Everyone is assigned to share Me with certain people. Try not to miss any more opportunities of people I send to you who have questions and need facts about Me. I send those whom you are equipped to share and serve.

Sometimes you are just a part of their journey to Me. Sometimes you are the entire journey. There are people who I created who want to know more about Me and because of their inquisitiveness, they will seek you for answers. You are to answer them. They will analyze those answers and eventually they will enter into relationship with Me. Some of you that I have created are not in tune to My voice and My ways. You are part of their learnings.

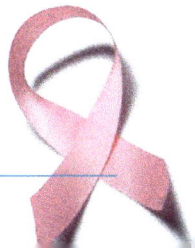

Exodus 16:6-8 (NIV) [6] So Moses and Aaron said to all the Israelites, "In the evening you will know that it was the LORD who brought you out of Egypt, [7] and in the morning you will see the glory of the LORD, because he has heard your grumbling against him. Who are we, that you should grumble against us?" [8] Moses also said, "You will know that it was the LORD when he gives you meat to eat in the evening and all the bread you want in the morning, because he has heard your grumbling against him. Who are we? You are not grumbling against us, but against the LORD."

I provide for you regardless of your attitude.

The you I created is different than who you are now. You have allowed the world to influence you in some very negative ways. Because of that worldly influence, you have adopted a negative attitude, which is somewhat hard to provide for and help.

That grumbling and complaining is unnecessary and quarrelsome and disrespectful to Me. You grumble as if My provisions mean nothing: you cannot save yourself. You cannot save yourself. I made you in My likeness and My image. You do not understand My calling on your life. You neglect the prayers you have prayed and the blessings which you have requested, which I answered and provided. You have difficulties to grow and to develop an appreciation for Me and what you are able to see what I do.

You are most ungrateful. Otherwise, your appreciation is brief and temporary. You do not understand your overall role, which makes it difficult to move forward without this disdain you exhibit when it is convenient for you.

Be still because I am God.

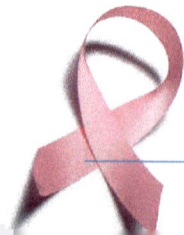

Exodus 20:1-2 (NIV) [1]And God spoke all these words: [2]"I am the LORD your God, who brought you out of Egypt, out of the land of slavery.

I bring you out of your troubles.

I bring you out of your troubles. I shed light on your dark places. I keep watch over you when you are in enemy territory and when the enemy is present. I provide boundaries when the enemy asks to sift you.

Your troubles would like to infect you and to overtake you and to emotionally harm you. Your troubles are designed to trouble you, and I allow those troubles in order to grow you up and strengthen you, to give you insight and to teach you how to live in spite of your trouble. I do not let those troubles overtake you.

Your troubles can be overcome because I hold you up while your troubles exist around you. Your troubles are temporary. I use everything to drive you back to Me! Your troubles should drive you to your knees and close the gap between us. Your troubles should not drive you to sin with your 'go-to's.' Your troubles, how to handle those troubles, and how those troubles come to resolve build your character. I want to build your character so that I can trust you with the ideals closest to My heart. I am committed to bring you out of your troubles. You will come out of those troubles stronger, and by design more focused on Me.

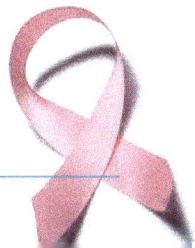

Leviticus 19:18 (NIV) [18] "'Do not seek revenge or bear a grudge against anyone among your people, but love your neighbor as yourself. I am the LORD.

Do not hold a grudge and love one another.

This cannot be that hard. I love you in spite of what you do. I already know what happened. I knew what happened before it happened. I knew your response as well. What most disappointed Me was that I loved you through that attack on your character and that insult on your person, that theft and that injustice and that terrible family member who hurt you. My love is supposed to lift you. My love should elevate your spirit and soul. My love closes gaps and bridges divides. My love defines you and defies the status quo. My love creates a giving spirit. My love moves you to a better place—one where you forgive and move on. I am working on the other person, too. Sometimes that other person is you.

My love is enough for you. I love you enough for you to love yourself and others. I love you enough for you to be overwhelmed and influenced to love others, especially those who harm you. Why don't you love yourself? I sill love you. Forgive yourself. Love yourself again. You not loving yourself is stopping you from loving others, and sometimes loving Me.

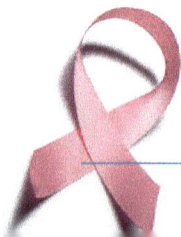

John 13:14-15 (NIV) [14] Now that I, your Lord and Teacher, have washed your feet, you also should wash one another's feet. [15] I have set you an example that you should do as I have done for you.

I have prepared you as an example.

When Jesus washes the disciple's feet, they are overwhelmed as are you when I do things for you. The foot washing was symbolic of the lengths We will go for you to show you Our love and service. We do this demonstration so that you can love and serve others. I am preparing you to serve others daily. You may not get a warning for the need to save someone, so you need to pay close attention to My lessons and demonstrations.

When you are called to serve someone, you cannot refuse. You want to be ready. I am certain that this could be overwhelming but you are prepared! Stop what you are doing. Listen to the person in front of you. Bring their burdens and concerns to Me in prayer with them present, where they can hear you pray to Me on their behalf. Then ask them how you can help, then take action on what they say. Give it to them as I have blessed you to give.

I choose you to serve others. The blessings I give to you are to be shared. You are an example which starts with sharing your blessings. I did not bless you to be selfish. I blessed you to bless others.

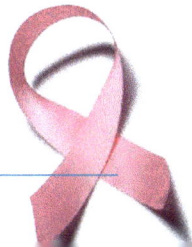

Matthew 5:14-16 (NIV) [14] "You are the light of the world. A town built on a hill cannot be hidden. [15] Neither do people light a lamp and put it under a bowl. Instead they put it on its stand, and it gives light to everyone in the house. [16] In the same way, let your light shine before others, that they may see your good deeds and glorify your Father in heaven.

Be the light I created you to be.

Light is defined as you living correctly and with truth. As light, you are to pray and be optimistic. You are to shed love on their situations. As light, your words should be uplifting and not gossiping. You should pray and not pass judgement. Light means you talk about Me and My word.

Light means that you love and listen and lead according to My word. I created you to be light in this world. This world needs light and I chose you. I chose you because I know that I can trust you with My message. I am in need of everyone keeping their focus on the goal—keeping peace within the world.

Stop trying to be part of the world. They don't even like you. You don't fit in either. As soon as you open your mouth, they know you don't belong to them. If you would just be the light then you can do My work, instead of trying to disguise My light as shade, or otherwise.

Stop trying to pretend that you don't belong to Me. They all see through that act: Your light is shining through the disguise.

Use your light to bring others to Me. Use light to influence the darkness that you encounter. I am with you.

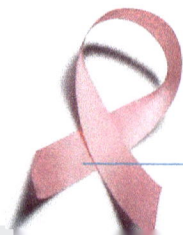

1 Peter 5:5-6 (NIV) [5] In the same way, you who are younger, submit yourselves to your elders. All of you, clothe yourselves with humility toward one another, because, "God opposes the proud but shows favor to the humble." [6] Humble yourselves, therefore, under God's mighty hand, that he may lift you up in due time.

I will remind you to be humble.

Humbleness and humility are characteristics that I require and deem worthy of fear. When you are humble, I am pleased. You are My child, My creation, My best work—but so is everyone and everything else. I created everything and everyone, so nobody is better than anyone else.

Humbleness is priceless and keeps you whole. I want you humble because you will be able to hear Me. The other point is that if you are humble, I can still count on you to work and show up when I call. Lacking humbleness may mean that you miss the next assignment.

I will remind you to be humble. This reminder is not going to be repeated. My attitude which that you should remember the instructions I gave you about humbleness, which is synonymous to meekness. I am consumed with your character because you were made in My image, which means you behave like Me, as well as look like Me.

Humble is what Jesus is. It is what Paul is. Sometimes it was not Peter, but these are the words I gave Peter and that is a characteristic that he can exhibit. So can you. Humble.

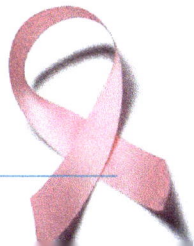

Numbers 6:24-26 (NIV) [24] """The LORD bless you and keep you; [25] the LORD make his face shine on you and be gracious to you; [26] the LORD turn his face toward you and give you peace.'"

I am your God.

I bless you, despite your inability to deserve My blessings. I keep you from hurt, harm and danger. I keep you from sin. I keep you from harming yourself.

I turn My face toward and smile upon you. I smile at you. I smile at you and your antics and your jokes and your pleas. Sometimes I just smile. I make My face shine upon you by providing My favor and giving you the desires of your heart.

I am gracious unto you, forgiving you, and loving you unconditionally.

I am facing you so that I can see and hear you so that you know that I am attentive to you and your voice and needs.

I give you peace. Peace. Peace that you ask for and desperately need to sleep at night, to stop smoking, overeating, and drinking. Peace that I provide stays and is not moved by outward situations. Peace that keeps you whole. I give you My peace—not peace that can be purchased or boxed or bought.

Bless you! I bless you!

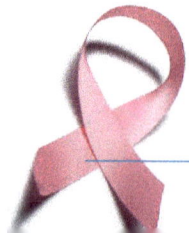

Psalm 8:1 (KJV) O LORD, our Lord, how excellent is thy name in all the earth! who hast set thy glory above the heavens.

I am your Lord.

When I hear this verse, I am moved. You have called on Me in a most reverent manner. I am considerate of you, so you should feel the rest I have given you when you utter these words.

When you get frightened and afraid and anxious, utter those words, so that I can give you some peace and some mental rest. You are worried and overwhelmed, but when you utter those words, you are surrounded by peace; you are overcome by an awesome breeze of relief. Realize that I am that breeze, that relief, that portion of strength, and that refreshing.

When you honor Me with those words of honor and adoration, you are releasing mental toxins that have previously prevented you from worshipping Me.

I am particular to the first four words. When you say 'O Lord' to get My attention, you say it with so much reverence, which makes Me attentive to your voice. When you say 'our Lord,' you have claimed Me as your Lord and God. That claim is mutual—you were already Mine; I made you.

Keep adoring Me and keep focusing on Me so I can clear the area around your heart. I want to infuse it with love so that you can love again.

I like the reverence in your voice which was produced by the reverence in your heart.

My love and My child, I will bless you. Relax.

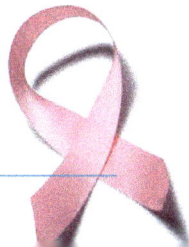

Psalm 19:14 (NIV) [14] May these words of my mouth and this meditation of my heart be pleasing in your sight, LORD, my Rock and my Redeemer.

I do want your mouth and heart to please Me.

Well, you do not always speak well—you say amazing things to others, making them less than whole. Your mouth can be dangerous. That is unhealthy and cruel. We need to use your mouth to encourage others –that will please Me. Remove that negative talk to yourself and others. I taught you that there is power in your tongue. So many of your words could lift but they lower the other person.

I send people to you to say positive words to you, so therefore I send you to people to say positive words to them. For that reason, you need to be sensitive as to why people are in your presence. Why did I send them to you? Why did I send you to them? You meet people because I orchestrate that meeting between you and others for My glory and purpose.

Your heart is Mine. It belongs to Me! I cannot tell you that enough so that you can stop ignoring Me so that your heart does not have to be broken. I am considering the meditation of your heart.

I am encouraging you to seek Me when you want to say something ugly or false or disparaging or shallow or rude or simply lame. Seek Me. Cry out to Me. I am listening. I am waiting on you to share your burdens with Me.

Your mouth is the place where My words come from. Your mouth is where My praise comes from. Out of that same mouth you hurl insults. There is confusion in that. It is hard for others to listen if you do both.

I want the meditation of your heart to be on Me, your Rock and your Redeemer. That is awesome claim of Me. For that, you should share Me with others.

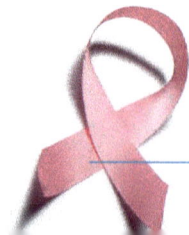

Psalm 119:11(NIV) [11] I have hidden your word in my heart that I might not sin against you.

I am proud that My word is in your heart.

Is My word inside of you? Can My word come out of you with clarity and understanding? Can you share My word with others? Will you tell someone that I saved you? Will you tell someone that I will save them? Can you use My word to find comfort and peace? Can you use My word to determine love, and it's opposite, indifference? Do you know My word in a manner that allows others to seek Me?

I gave you the Bible as the Instruction Manual. So many of you use it sparingly but have many needs that would be solved by reading My word. If you read it and pray that I share with you understanding and wisdom, then when you need saving in your time of trouble, you can easily repeat and consider My word, which will offer you the peace you desire.

When you know My word, sinning should be less. I know that some of you sin willfully, but you will still know My word at least know that you are wrong and will be at least know that you are wrong and will be driven to respond in remorse.

I offer you the Holy Spirit to indwell within you. The choices yours but My word should influence you to avoid sin so that you will not be subject to My consequences.

If My word is within you, then your behavior and words and deeds and thoughts and attitude should reflect our relationship and your study effort.

Keep reading. Keep studying. You may have to read it several times. Don't get nervous. Don't be afraid.

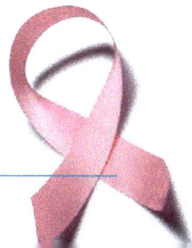

Psalm 139:14 (NIV) [14] I praise you because I am fearfully and wonderfully made; your works are wonderful, I know that full well.

I made you.

Yes, I made you! I made you and have plans for you. I am showing you My will and direction daily. I did a good job on you. You are My best work. I need you to understand that you are so critical of yourself, but why? You are fearfully and wonderfully made! I made you!

I am still sure that I made you on purpose because you have a purpose—a purpose I predestined for you.

I made you so that you could do My work. I know that you know it but you sometimes act like you don't know.

I need you to have confidence that I have instilled within you. You have allowed the world to challenge your confidence and your character. You have yielded to them in ways that you never yield to Me.

Daughter, please stop doubting your abilities to serve Me through who I made you to be. You are fearfully and wonderfully made. I know because I made you. I made you to do great things, to accomplish great works, and to be a major force for Me.

Go for it! Go confidently in who I made you to be and what I created you to do. Behave in such a manner that the world distances itself from you.

I am the Lord, your God!

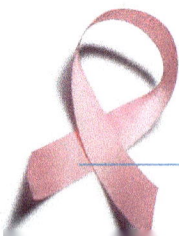

Proverbs 3:5-6 (NIV) [5] Trust in the LORD with all your heart and lean not on your own understanding; [6] in all your ways submit to Him, and He will make your paths straight.

Trust Me, and only Me.

I don't think I need to keep explaining this because wisdom dictates you would remember where wisdom comes from and how wisdom is given and what you should be doing.

I said for you not to lean on your own understanding because your thoughts have not been close enough to Me. Your thoughts have been tainted and drawn away from Me. So when I say seek Me, I really mean that. I need to share new revelations with you all the time, but it is difficult to get your attention at times. You are listening to others, sometimes causing you to question Me and My sovereignty and grace, mercy and forgiveness. They have a powerful enough voice and powerful enough influence that you have distanced yourself from Me to accommodate them and to impress them and to be accepted by them. Why do you exchange Me for yet someone else I created? I can only imagine how you thought that would be okay—it is your need of wisdom.

Trust. Trust Me. Trust Me with all you heart. Trust Me with the parts that you have previously kept from Me. You have partitioned your heart so it is hard to trust Me with all your heart when your heart is preoccupied. I have your best interest in mind because you represent Me. You are a reflection of Me.

Trust.

Lean.

Submit.

To Me.

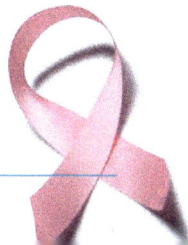

Proverbs 23:7a (KJV) [7] For so as a man thinketh in his heart, so is he

I am concerned about your thoughts. Most of them do not include Me.

What you think is who you are. What you think about dictates your character. What you think about dictates your actions. What you think about dictates your mood and attitude. What you think about determines your friends. What you think about determines your success at work. Your thoughts control what you do, what you dream about, and what you consider important.

What are you thinking about? Why are you thinking about that? Will your thought pleas me or bring glory to My name? on the contrary, will y our thoughts cause Me to be angry and upset? Will your thoughts cause My reputation to be questioned? Will your thoughts cause people to question your love of Me? Will your thoughts cause others to question whether you are a Christian?

Are your thoughts powerful enough to cause you to sin? Are your thoughts strong enough to cause you to avoid sin? Are your thoughts influential enough to stop sinning? You are not sure really, but if you answered no to any of those questions, you can then guarantee that you NEED Me.

I created you with a self-esteem which should sustain the thoughts which cause you to question why should you sin. Your thoughts can bring love to My name.

Think about Me so that you can be more like Me, understand Me and My ways and My will, and believe in Me with an increased faith.

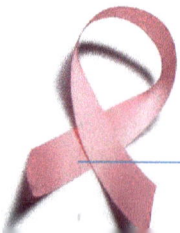

Habakkuk 2:2 (KJV) [2] And the LORD answered me, and said, Write the vision, and make it plain upon tables, that he may run that readeth it.

Vision starts with Me.

Vision is an interesting word. I know because I created the concept then provided millions of examples . . . daily.

The vision I speak of begins with Me. The problem you are having is because you do not seek My will when you create that vision. Effective and lasting vision comes from Me and is centered on My word and will. This is the only way that you will see that vision come to pass.

A vision that I can bless embodies the use of the gifts that I have given you to share with others as I have commanded you.

A great vision honors Me and represents My will. A great vision keeps Me first and is one where you ask My permission rather than ask for Me to bless what you already put together.

My vision for you needs to be adopted and adapted and managed. My vision is what will happen.

How close is what you want to what I want? What I want and will is what will prevail. When you write that vision, I am revealing My will—pay attention.

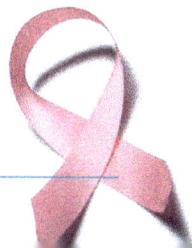

Matthew 14:31(NIV) [31] Immediately, Jesus reached out His hand and caught him. "You of little faith," He said, "why did you doubt?"

Your doubt is offensive and counterproductive.

Daughter, why do you doubt Me? Didn't I show you that that issue before it grew too big for treatment? Didn't I stop your child from dying? Didn't I keep your finances from falling when you would have had to spend all of your money on treatment? Didn't I save your daughter?

Daughter, you are supposed to have faith in My abilities, My grace, My mercy, My love and My timing. What does it really take for you to be faithful? I mean you weren't in that building that was bombed, where hundreds died but you were home on the couch . . . against your will, but totally within My will. I caused that plane to leave late which caused you to miss the missile attack. I caused your bus tour to stop because there was a bomb around the next corner. You returned home unscathed. You looked at the news and realized that you could have been dead or injured.

I save you from events and catastrophic issues which you will never connect to Me, but it was Me.

When I show you what I saved you from, it is designed to increase your faith; faith which exhibits your trust and love for Me. When you have a whimsical faith or complete doubt prevails, I am offended.

I have given you no reason to doubt Me, so stop it!

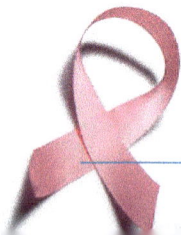

Deuteronomy 6:5 (NIV) [5] Love the LORD your God with all your heart and with all your soul and with all your strength.

I deserve your love—all of it!

The love I expect and anticipate is the love which you give for no reason. I love you even when you sin. You love Me until you sin. When you sin, you quit loving Me.

I really hope that changes soon. Your love cannot be conditional when I am the very reason that you exist. Sometimes you treat Me like others. I am quite different and I actually deserve your love.

You 'love' others who do nothing for you and quite possibly do not even like you, but your love for Me can be lukewarm. Not sure how you have managed to justify that action.

Love Me with all of yourself. Don't hold any love back. Don't be selfish. Don't stop loving for any reason.

I love you, too! I know that as the provider of your love, I give you more than enough for you to love Me completely, love yourself, and to love others as I have defined and commanded.

Stop loving like you are going to run out. That is impossible. I am the Replenisher of your love.

Love.

Love extravagantly.

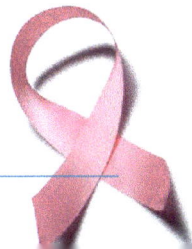

John 11:35 (NIV) [35] Jesus wept.

I love His compassion.

Jesus was ministering far away when Lazarus dies. With My consent and provision, Jesus returns to raise Lazarus from the dead. But before He raises Lazarus, Jesus wept. Jesus cried. You are afraid to cry. You think that it makes you weak but the compassion that your tears convey are powerful.

I like the compassion which you convey when you cry for others and their situations. I assigned you to be compassionate and when you do, your behavior makes Me proud.

Jesus already knew that He would be raising Lazarus and cried anyway.

What do you find important enough to be compassionate about? Who gets close enough to earn your compassion?

Compassion and your exhibit thereof aligns you to Me. Compassion makes you like Me. Keep focused on Me when determining how to be compassionate and to whom. I will guide your head, heart and hand.

I know how efficient you want to be and I know that compassion requires time that you don't think that you have. But this is My will.

Compassion reminds My people when they feel it from you that I am still God.

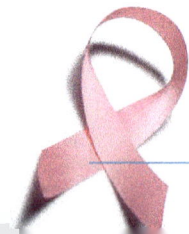

Romans 8:26 (NIV) [26] In the same way, the Spirit helps us in our weakness. We do not know what we ought to pray for, but the Spirit himself intercedes for us through wordless groans.

I gave you the Holy Spirit.

You get discouraged and frustrated because you took a wrong turn or you experienced a misstep. Take heart. I am right here!

I sent you the Holy Spirit! You NEED the Holy Spirit which knows My will and the Holy Spirit will intercede for you to Me. You NEED the Holy Spirit!

You are weak! You fold under the slightest amount of pressure. That layoff was not supposed to be detrimental or show stopping. That miscarriage was not the end of the world. Your husband cheating was not the end of your life. You recovered from bad credit. You got degrees that you never intended. You have achieved the things that people said you never would.

I love you! I have not left you or abandoned you. You are My daughter! I take care of you. Everyday. In all conditions. Under all conditions. Without condition. No strings attached.

Prayer helps our relationship. Stop avoiding Me. Stop avoiding My voice. Stop avoiding My words. Stop avoiding Me.

Stop using the excuse of not knowing what to say to Me. I just want you to talk to Me. Tell Me everything! I know that you can't tell Me everything because you are ashamed. You should not have done something that you could not share with Me.

Just pray.

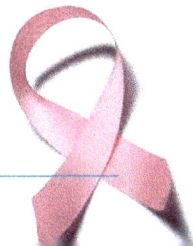

Romans 8:27 (NIV) [27] And he who searches our hearts knows the mind of the Spirit, because the Spirit intercedes for God's people in accordance with the will of God.

I search your heart; it belongs to Me.

I search your heart: yes, I do. I have given the Holy Spirit that authority as well. I need to know what you are feeling and your intentions both of which come from your heart.

I have to protect your heart from those elements which cause your heart to be distanced from Me.

Our searches align with the mind in such a manner, that the Spirit knows what I need to know about your state of mind and emotion.

That information causes Me to provoke the Intercessor to start to pray for you. You need an intercessor because you are distracted and distanced from Me, your calling, your gifts, talents, and even your responsibilities. That intercessor knows My will.

I need you to be focused on Me and My word and My will.

Daughter, I love you and I want you to have the desires of your heart based on My will. My will protects you and keeps you whole. My will loves you and holds you together. Your Intercessor is assigned to you. I know it because I assigned the Intercessor to you.

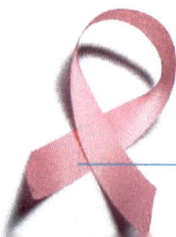

Romans 8:28 (NIV) [28] And we know that in all things God works for the good of those who love Him, who have been called according to His purpose.

I am in ALL things.

In ALL things . . . I am in ALL things, first of all. I am a part of everything that you are doing and that you want to do and that I have assigned you to do.

I know that you often look your situation and wonder where I am, but I promise I am right here, especially when it feels like I am not.

I have all details working together for your good. Do you remember when you missed that accident when you left home late? You did get to work to late but when you arrived, you were told that the meeting had been moved back one hour.

Look at the events that happen and the details which surround your life more carefully to discern whether you can see how even the worst of details can come together for your good. These events move you back to My will.

Loving Me is part of the contingent details but loving Me is what you do most of the time. The last part is being called according to My purpose. You are called for My purposes. I have a plan, a will, a design, and an outcome. For everyone I created. I am focused on each detail. So even when it does not look or feel like you are making progress, I am making progress for you and your situation.

ALL.

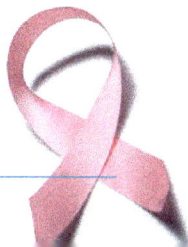

Romans 8:29-30 (NIV) [29] For those God foreknew He also predestined to be conformed to the image of His Son, that He might be the firstborn among many brothers and sisters. [30] And those He predestined, He also called; those He called, He also justified; those He justified, He also glorified.

I am in control.

When I sent My Son to die because of global sin, I made a decision. That decision saved generations present and future for generations to come.

I created you in Our image, Our likeness, and because of that you are supposed to be closely aligned to Us.

I predestined you.

I called you.

I justified you.

I glorified you.

I predestined you to be like Jesus and to My will. I have an image of you and I really want you to be closer to My image.

I created you.

I called you to carry out My purpose and My will. I picked this calling especially for you. I picked you because I created you for this calling.

I justified you and reconciled you to Myself. I forgive you for your sins, even those directly against Me, and love you in spite of your shortcomings, issues and doubts. I only bring you closer to My bosom because you are My daughter.

I glorified you. I dust off the dirt that others want to pile on you and throw at you and soil you with. I clean you up. I erase your past, parts of your present, and portions of your future.

I am your God.

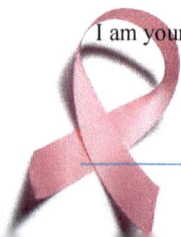

Romans 8:31 (NIV) [31] What, then, shall we say in response to these things? If God is for us, who can be against us?

I am for you.

Daughter. Do not start making a list! I am not interested in your list. I know all of your enemies, actual and perceived.

I am for you! I am your creator! I am a fan. I keep you close to My heart and on My mind. I know My love for you causes you trouble with others I have created. I am still in charge. My Will will still be done. No exceptions. I know that living your life for Me is not popular, uncomfortable, challenging, and overall intimidating.

There will be many people that do not want you to be successful or accomplished or happy or excited or loving or kind or dedicated to My work or committed to My word. They would prefer your misery and your attitude and your bitterness to develop and prevail.

I am for you. While I know that you do not seek My approval first, I'm the Only One that matters.

My approval is the Only One that counts toward your self-esteem and self-image and self-worth.

I love you and I always will.

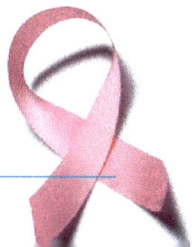

Romans 8:35 (NIV) [35] Who shall separate us from the love of Christ? Shall trouble or hardship or persecution or famine or nakedness or danger or sword?

I cannot be separated from you.

Who can take you away from Me? I am your God. What can take you from Me? I am your God. I created you. I invest in you each second of your life because of My plans for you.

No, I am working on it so that you stop considering that as an option.

Trouble. Hardship. Persecution. Famine. Nakedness. Danger. Sword.

Trouble is going to come your way. I am your God who saves you and keeps you. Trouble strengthens you. You survived and was better because of it.

Hardship will come and go but I will always be your God. I pull you through hardships. I provide during hardships.

Persecution is just what others think they can distract you with, inclusive of character flaws. I am still here and others have certainly abandoned you.

Famine has not overtaken you. I know it was hard. You thought it was personal. It was. I need you to experience some things that you to see and experience so that you can help others.

Nakedness had never quite been an issue—not a real one.

Danger is certainly imminent, however, you have My protection, which I keep really tight.

Sword—no sword has overcome you. I won't let it.

Nothing can separate you from My love unless I consent. Don't anticipate it.

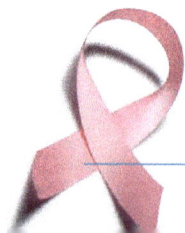

Colossians 3:23 (NIV) [23] Whatever you do, work at it with all your heart, as working for the Lord, not for human masters,

I am taking note of your work ethic.

The work, all of it, that you do is for Me. Don't get emotional when others criticize you and your performance. Just keep working for Me. Do your best as if I am personally inspecting each step. Because I am.

Your work ethic is your character. That character is My creation. My children make Me look good or bad—never in between. Your work ethic lets Me know that I can trust you. I have big plans for you, but I need you to be ready.

What others say really does not mean anything. Stop worrying about it. Learn to ignore that as noise.

Remind yourself when you get discouraged that I am the reason you have that position at that company at this time. I am the reason and you will just maintain what I have already assigned you to do.

Your work ethic means that you believe in Me and you recognize me as the God that I am.

Let Me be your center such that the noise around you is avoidable and non-influential. Give Me all that you are and all that you have.

That work ethic is a report card of hope you feel about Me.

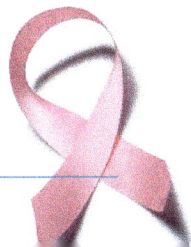

1 Thessalonians 5:17 (NIV) [17] pray continually

I expect you to pray.

Two simple words: pray continually. You have asked several times how to do this and why is that necessary.

The how is simple: pray in all situations. Before you eat. Before you drive. When you arrive. When you get good news. When you get bad news. When you achieve a goal. When you don't. When you are happy. When you are sad. When you cannot breathe. When you are depressed. When you are angry. Or bitter. Or broken. Or battered. Or heartbroken. Or depleted. Or famished. Or confused. And counterproductive.

When someone is mean to you. When someone forgives you. When someone hurts you. When someone bullies you. When someone protects you. When someone shares Jesus with you. When someone helps you.

You pray because I say to. Because Jesus taught you how to pray. Because Jesus prayed. Because Jesus prayed for you. Because I gave you the Holy Spirit.

Why do you need to pray all the time—you have asked a million times. Because prayer closes the gap between us. Because I talk during your prayer time. Because I listen to you. Because I reveal My will to you during prayer.

Because I said so.

Pray.

Continually.

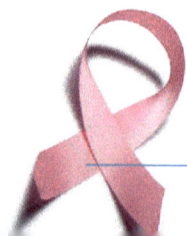

Jude 24-25 (KJV) [24] Now unto him that is able to keep you from falling, and to present you faultless before the presence of his glory with exceeding joy, [25] To the only wise God our Saviour, be glory and majesty, dominion and power, both now and ever. Amen.

I am wise and able.

I see you when you hear these words. You go the most spiritual place in your heart, mind, and soul where your worship is the most pure and authentic.

I love how these words return you to Me. These words invoke your worship and praise to Me.

The most important part of this verse is My message to you: I keep you from falling into sin.

I keep you faultless when I present you to Myself on My throne.

I am proud to keep you from falling into sin before My throne of grace with joy, exceedingly.

I am the only wise God.

I deserve your glory and majesty.

I am dominion and power.

I deserve it forever.

Of all the words I inspired, these words articulate the essence of Me and what I require and what you can expect and what you should want to give to Me.

I really do keep My word and keep My promises. Come closer to Me so I can fully do that for you.

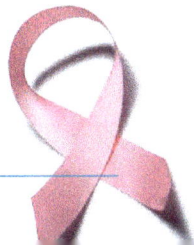

Revelation 3:16 (NIV) [16] So, because you are lukewarm—neither hot nor cold—I am about to spit you out of my mouth.

I will spit you out.

Daughter, absolutely pick a side! Make a decision! Just one! Right now. Remain consistent with that decision. When you don't choose, you are trying to please too many people.

Make a decision. You have the tools for making a decision. You go with the tide or the wind. That is not a stable location.

Lukewarm is not a good place. I don't want you close to Me. Lukewarm can be bought, bribed, and influenced. The power of that influence can change daily.

I would respect you for making a choice. Even if it fails.

Lukewarm cannot be trusted. It exhibits a lack of depth and character. I didn't create you like that. That is not in My image.

I cannot continue to support you in this matter. I have to spit you out, which means I will distance Myself from you until you choose and abandon that middle of the road, non-choosing, please everyone behavior.

Make a choice.

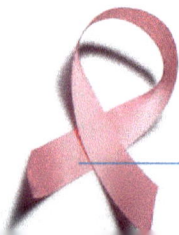

Hebrews 13:5b (NIV) ⁵ because God has said, "Never will I leave you; never will I forsake you."

I am not going to live you or abandon you.

I will never leave you nor will I ever forsake you. You have sinned to a level that when someone does what you have done already, you judge them, but I forgive you.

You have done some awful things, yet I am still here! I bless you. Daily. I blow breath in your lungs because I have a purpose for you.

I have not left and never will, while you deny Me. You act like I don't exist when you don't know how people will accept you because of Me. It is seriously offensive! But when you are struggling, you call Me first and expect Me to respond in real time, otherwise known as immediately.

Never will I forsake you. I will not desert you. I will not abandon you. I will not quit on you.

I will not trade you for something or someone else.

I know that everyone abandons you. Some of those people are supposed to leave—their season and time was up. They would cause more harm than good.

Just because 'they' abandoned you, does not mean that I will. They do not define Me; I define them.

Nor leave.

Nor forsake.

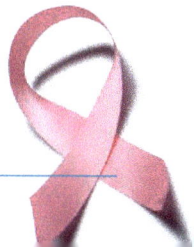

Romans 8:36-37 (NIV) [36] As it is written: "For your sake we face death all day long; we are considered as sheep to be slaughtered." [37] No, in all these things we are more than conquerors through Him who loved us.

You are more than conquerors.

You belong to Me. I know that you are at risk because of Me and My calling on your life and your purpose. I also know that I am your shield and protector. I block the enemies that desire to overtake you. I change your path such that you are not distracted by sin.

I am still in charge even when and especially because of your most severe adversity.

I made you strong. Resilient. Persistent. Dynamic. Audacious. Powerful. Kind. Loving. Charismatic. Profound. Mighty. Proud. Practical. Driven. Warm. Thoughtful. Strategic. Admirable. Respected. Respectful. Tenacious. Outstanding. Outlandish. Outrageous. Brilliant.

I made you ALL of this and more. I make you with these qualities because I need those qualities available when adversity comes. I cannot afford for you to fold.

You are a conqueror. More than a conqueror. That I made to overcome that parts of the world where I send you.

You are more than a conqueror because I love you. You are to conquer all that is counterproductive to Me, My will, My message, and My plan.

A conqueror.

More than.

For Me.

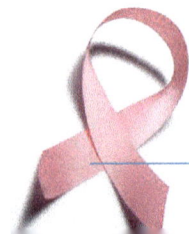

Romans 8:38-39 (NIV) [38] For I am convinced that neither death nor life, neither angels nor demons, neither the present nor the future, nor any powers, [39] neither height nor depth, nor anything else in all creation, will be able to separate us from the love of God that is in Christ Jesus our Lord.

Nothing can separate Us from each other.

When Paul penned these words, he was convinced of My love and its overwhelming power. It may have been because I saved him on the road to Damascus. Or maybe it was because I called him to preach in spite of his slanderous talk against me before I saved him.

Maybe it was the power that he understood My love to have once he was on the side of Jesus and now he was able to transform his previous followers to newly saved followers.

Whenever it was that Paul realized that My love conquers all, you should be close to realizing it as well.

I don't know what else I can do to convince you. I have done enough, more than enough, to show you the power of My love and the measure of My love.

I am the Lord, your God. I love you and I will not let anyone separate you from Me. You are Mine—you belong to Me. I may have let satan have limited access to Job and I may have let satan sift Peter and I may have let satan have limited access to you. Remember, My love makes satan ask for permission. My love requires that access to be limited. My love shuts that access down.

My love for you cannot be interrupted and we cannot be separated by anyone or anything without My consent.

The answer is No!

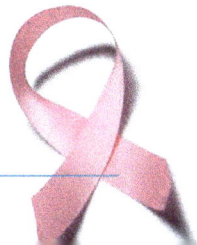

James 1:2-5 (NIV) [2] Consider it pure joy, my brothers and sisters, whenever you face trials of many kinds, [3] because you know that the testing of your faith produces perseverance. [4] Let perseverance finish its work so that you may be mature and complete, not lacking anything. [5] If any of you lacks wisdom, you should ask God, who gives generously to all without finding fault, and it will be given to you.

I know it is hard to consider having joy during trials but there is a reason why.

Joy during trials does not seem natural. The world dictates your battle face during your trials. I require joy because I am present and in control.

I allow trials to increase your faith through perseverance. If you never go through anything, then you will remain the same and never grow. These trials teach what reading can never do for you. You have to go through it so that you can mature.

During the trials, I give you wisdom because you asked. If you were not in a trial, then you would not have asked. But since you asked, I'll give it to you. Just ask.

I am training you to believe. You doubt because you have a memory—sometimes I wish I could wipe clean. I need you to want to believe—believe in Me.

Stop praying to be released from trials. I need you to survive those trials. I need you to persevere. It is required so that I can answer the rest of your prayers.

Keep your eyes on Me during trials. I am waiting to be your Only Source.

Trials are inevitable—they are coming. How you handle them is My concern.

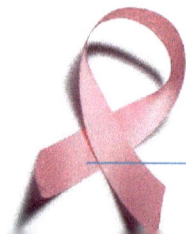

Luke 12:22-26 (NIV) [22] Then Jesus said to his disciples: "Therefore I tell you, do not worry about your life, what you will eat; or about your body, what you will wear. [23] For life is more than food, and the body more than clothes. [24] Consider the ravens: They do not sow or reap, they have no storeroom or barn; yet God feeds them. And how much more valuable you are than birds! [25] Who of you by worrying can add a single hour to your life? [26] Since you cannot do this very little thing, why do you worry about the rest?

Do not worry.

I wished and commanded you not to worry but you are simply disobedient. Food and clothes are material aspects of life but are not essential. They seem essential and worth worrying about but they are not. Have you ever been naked? I mean really naked without your choice. No, you have never been naked and unable to go in public. You may not have exactly what you want to wear but you will never be without clothes.

Maybe you were hungry for an extended period of time, but you will not be hungry forever. You will not be hungry until the point of death. There are people assigned to insure that you are fed. You may not have all that you want to eat or the food that you want but you are not hungry.

Your life and your body are most important. Your life serves Me. Your life witnesses for Me. Your life reflects Me. Your life is valuable to Me. Your life causes Me to bring others to Me. Your life is maintained by Me. Your body works for Me, so I feed it and clothe it. I manage its health and fitness.

If worry were valuable, it could add money to your accounts or add hours to your life or add value to your existence or worry could save you. But because it is not valuable, it cannot do any of those things.

So stop worrying.

That's time and money which you are wasting which you could be using for Me.

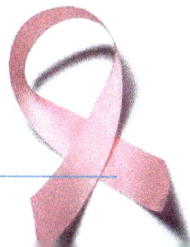

Luke 13:12-13 (NIV) [12] When Jesus saw her, He called her forward and said to her, "Woman, you are set free from your infirmity." [13] Then He put His hands on her, and immediately she straightened up and praised God.

Your faith has healed you.

Come close to Me so that you can hear Me call you to Myself so that I can heal you. Come close to Me so I can loose what had bound you for ever so long. When Jesus called her, she was close to Him, in the same building, but ultimately, she was close enough for Him to observe her. She was close enough to Him for Him to call her over to Him and even in her ill state, she could make it to Him.

When she did, He announced her healed and then He touched her as confirmation. When He called her, she did not ask, 'were you talking to me?' and looking right, left, then back. She did not doubt or question. She was healed because of her presence at the synagogue which was the evidence of her faith. Her faith healed her.

Have faith.

Show up. In unsuspecting places.

Answer Me when I call.

Seek Me.

Stop asking the questions which usually incite doubt.

Accept My healing as a gift.

Her infirmity moved Jesus to touch her to heal her but she had to get close enough to be touched.

Be that woman: come to Me to be healed, get close, don't doubt, and praise Us.

Then share your testimony.

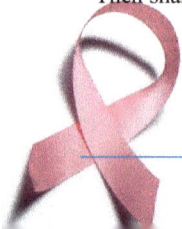

Luke 8:43-48 (NIV) [43] And a woman was there who had been subject to bleeding for twelve years, but no one could heal her. [44] She came up behind Him and touched the edge of His cloak, and immediately her bleeding stopped. [45] "Who touched me?" Jesus asked. When they all denied it, Peter said, "Master, the people are crowding and pressing against You." [46] But Jesus said, "Someone touched Me; I know that power has gone out from Me." [47] Then the woman, seeing that she could not go unnoticed, came trembling and fell at His feet. In the presence of all the people, she told why she had touched Him and how she had been instantly healed. [48] Then He said to her, "Daughter, your faith has healed you. Go in peace."

Exercise a faith that will impress Me.

Well finally someone picks Me amongst the many options for the solution for their situation that only I am available to fix, solve and solution. Only Me. That is what happens daily. You seek someone else to fix only what I can.

I only let some things be solved by others, virtually giving away My deserved glory, but in this case and other cases where I want there to be no doubt. I only allow the answer to come from Me. This is one such instance. I invite you to do something outrageous in order to seek Me, be healed, and show others that I am real and that you believe!

You have the same outrageous and outlandish spirit that she has and you can pursue Me that same way in your area of weakness. Take a risk on Me. I take a risk on you every day. I risk you daily.

I am your healer and I want to heal you. I am your strong tower. When she touched Him, she took the risk but she also reaped the reward. The reward was a long time coming. She considered the risk worth the reward.

I am glad she learned to trust. I hope you learn too, as well.

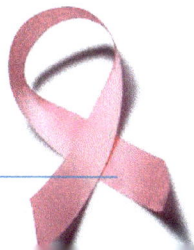

Ephesians 3:20 (KJV)—21(NIV) [20] Now unto him that is able to do exceeding abundantly above all that we ask or think, according to the power that worketh in us, [21] to him be glory in the church and in Christ Jesus throughout all generations, for ever and ever! Amen.

I can amaze you. I do it every day.

Again Paul shares his love for Me in an incredible and powerful manner. This is dedication from a contrite heart; one I have groomed incredibly and with such a level of detail that I cannot believe Myself where he has come from. I am certain that I dwell within him. I need to be certain that I dwell within you.

I do want to access the power I have embedded within you. You do not access that power. It lies dormant, unaccessed, and unused. This is not as designed. I designed you to operate with power. That power fuels the rest. If you do not access, use or believe that power, then I cannot do anything additional for you.

I am trying to awaken that power within you but you keep making excuses and avoiding Me. You make excuses for not accessing the power. You have the power I gave you but you have to access it, use it and believe in it. This is a mechanism to worship and praise Me.

One of My daughters even mixes the versions when she repeats this verse because and when she says the verse she closes her eyes and says it with such reverence. I appreciate her respect.

Access the power so you can see the exceeding abundance of what I can do, above all that you ask or think.

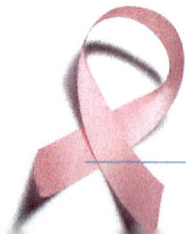

Ephesians 3:16-17 (NIV) [16] I pray that out of His glorious riches he may strengthen you with power through His Spirit in your inner being, [17] so that Christ may dwell in your hearts through faith. And I pray that you, being rooted and established in love,

I give you power.

When Paul prays for the Ephesians, and now you, he spends several verses praying about what means the most to Me.

When I had Paul pen these words, I did so with the intention of you to understand who I am. I planted the Holy Spirit in your inner being. With that inner being, you should easily submit yourself to Me. You can easily access the Holy Spirit for the power that I give as well as the reason why I give you that power: to use in My name, to advance My kingdom.

If I give you enough, then I will let you know what I am capable of. I need you to do all that you can so that you can know your maximum. I want your heart.

As your God, I want to know that I have your heart. I want you to tell others that I have your heart. I want others to see that your heart belongs to Me. And Me alone.

I have given you all the tools but you won't open the kit.

Access the Holy Spirit.

Access the power I provide.

Give Me full access to your heart.

Have faith.

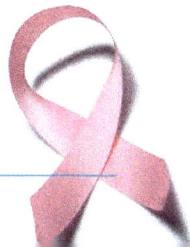

1 Samuel 16:7 (NIV) [7] But the LORD said to Samuel, "Do not consider his appearance or his height, for I have rejected him. The LORD does not look at the things people look at. People look at the outward appearance, but the LORD looks at the heart."

I look at your heart.

Why would I be impressed with an outward appearance that I created? I created that handsome creature. I am not impressed with what I did on purpose.

His heart will impress Me, though, because the world has tainted the pure heart which I created. I am sure that you did not mean to let the world influence you to harden your heart. Especially away from Me.

But when I sent Samuel to look at David to select him as king of Israel, I knew the depth and details of his heart. I know the depth and details of your heart.

I want others to be able to see your heart and I want you to be comfortable with the goodness of your heart. I want that heart to be available to Me. I don't want you to compromise the goodness of your heart in order to impress someone who is not a part of My will for you.

Look for the good in yourself and others by measure of the heart and nothing else. Your heart is what drives you. Your heart is what you use to stay motivated. Your heart is where your passion lives. Your heart causes you to believe. Your heart responds in real time.

Your heart belongs to Me.

So give it back.

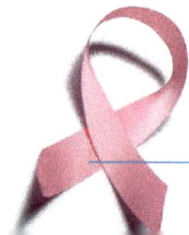

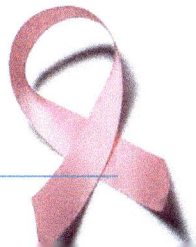

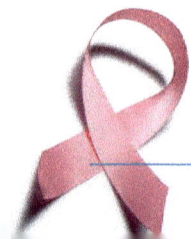

Index

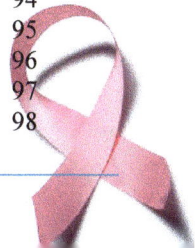

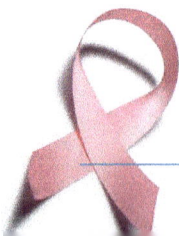

Acknowledgements

God, thank You for Your plans for me. Thank You for ***Her Story: The Legacy of Her Fight, The Devotional,*** and choosing me to complete Your project. I just want to please You, God. Thank You for continuing to anoint me and to invest in me and my gifts, which keep surprising me. Thank You for loving and forgiving me.

Hillary and Nehemiah, thank you for supporting me and my endeavors. Thank you for loving me, especially when I do nothing without a pen and a clipboard, thank you for enduring my late nights, your ideas, the sounding board, the love and the support. Thank you for celebrating our legacy.

To my prayer partners and to my accountability partners, thank you for the long talks and the powerful prayers and the encouragement.

To the readers who this will reach and empower and touch and affect, may these words empower you and help you reach some resolve. May you be inspired to achieve your goals and dreams. May you enhance your relationship with God so that your other relationships will also improve. May you enhance your self-esteem through prayer and study. May you have courage and peace. Share love the best you can until you can share love without reservation.

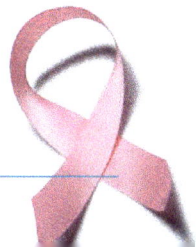

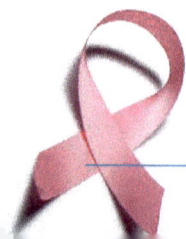

About the Advocate

The author believes these devotionals will help you to grow and create the study life that you and God both deserve.

Do not hesitate to ask, to engage at a high level of participation, anticipating God's best for you!

@onediangage (twitter) ♦ onediagage@onediagage.com ♦ facebook.com/onediagageministries

youtube.com/onediagage ♦ blogtalkradio.com/onediagage ♦ ongage (Instagram)

www.onediagage.com

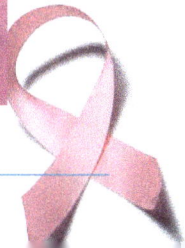

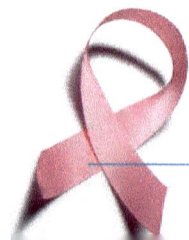

PREACHER ♦ ADVOCATE ♦ TEACHER ♦ FACILITATOR

CONFERENCE SPEAKER ♦ PANELIST ♦ WORKSHOP LEADER

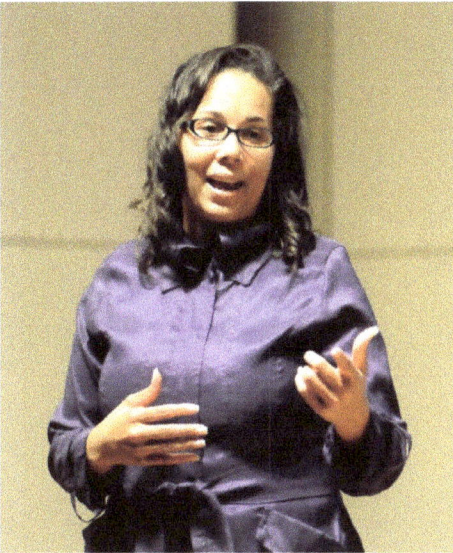

To invite Ms. Gage to speak at your church, women's ministry, breast cancer awareness groups, Or other ministry.

Please contact us at: www.onedigage.com

@onediangage (twitter) ♦ onediagage@onediagage.com ♦ facebook.com/onediagageministries

youtube.com/onediagage ♦ blogtalkradio.com/onediagage ♦ ongage (Instagram)

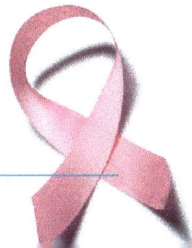

Her Story
121

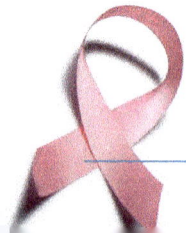

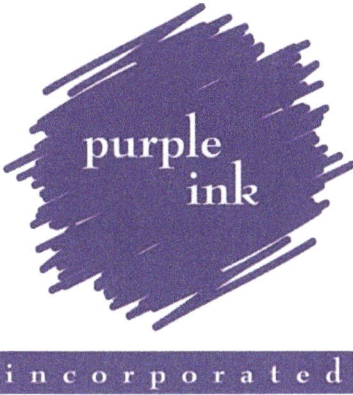

Publishing

Do you have a book you want to write, but do not know what to do?

Do you have a book you need to publish but do not know how to start?

Would publishing move your career forward?

Let us help

onediagage@purpleink.net ♦ www.purpleink.net

713.705.5530 ♦ 512.715.4243

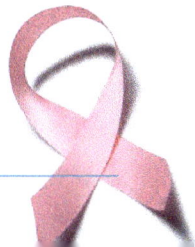

www.ingramcontent.com/pod-product-compliance
Lightning Source LLC
Chambersburg PA
CBHW071234020426
42333CB00015B/1468